Chemical Warrior

Hamish de Bretton-Gordon

Chemical Warrior

Syria, Salisbury and Saving Lives at War

HEADLINE

First published in 2020 by
HEADLINE PUBLISHING GROUP

1

Cataloguing in Publication Data is available from the British Library

Hardback ISBN 9781472274540
Trade paperback ISBN 9781472274557

Designed and typeset by EM&EN
Printed and bound in Great Britain by Clays Ltd, Elcograf S.p.A.

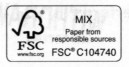

HEADLINE PUBLISHING GROUP
An Hachette UK Company
Carmelite House
50 Victoria Embankment
London EC4Y 0DZ

www.headline.co.uk
www.hachette.co.uk

Author's note

For reasons of national security and/or confidentiality, it has been necessary to change some details of events, including names, places and dates, when writing this book.

To the Syrian people.

May God give you a better tomorrow.

Contents

'Dulce et Decorum Est' – Wilfred Owen xi

Introduction 1

Part One – 'Men Marched Asleep'

1. Break up 13

2. New Assignment 25

3. The First Step 40

4. Anthrax 55

5. The Bomb 72

6. Convictions 96

7. New Beginnings 111

8. Sudden Death 124

Part Two – 'Like a Man in Fire'

9. The Arab Spring 139

10. A First Attempt 148

11. The Task Force 163

12. Crossing the Red Line 177

13. Getting a Sample 191

14. Harsh Reality 214

15. Breakdown and Breakthrough 225

Part Three – 'On Innocent Tongues'

16. Full Circle 243

17. Salisbury 254

18. Bending the Rules 273

19. The Future 282

Appendix: Surviving a Chemical or Biological Attack 293

Acknowledgements 303

'Dulce et Decorum Est'

Bent double, like old beggars under sacks,
Knock-kneed, coughing like hags, we cursed
   through sludge,
Till on the haunting flares we turned our backs,
And towards our distant rest began to trudge.
Men marched asleep. Many had lost their boots,
But limped on, blood-shod. All went lame; all blind;
Drunk with fatigue; deaf even to the hoots
Of gas-shells dropping softly behind.

Gas! GAS! Quick, boys!—An ecstasy of fumbling
Fitting the clumsy helmets just in time,
But someone still was yelling out and stumbling
And flound'ring like a man in fire or lime.—
Dim through the misty panes and thick green light,
As under a green sea, I saw him drowning.

In all my dreams before my helpless sight,
He plunges at me, guttering, choking, drowning.

If in some smothering dreams, you too could pace
Behind the wagon that we flung him in,

And watch the white eyes writhing in his face,
His hanging face, like a devil's sick of sin;
If you could hear, at every jolt, the blood
Come gargling from the froth-corrupted lungs,
Obscene as cancer, bitter as the cud
Of vile, incurable sores on innocent tongues,—
My friend, you would not tell with such high zest
To children ardent for some desperate glory,
The old Lie: *Dulce et decorum est
Pro patria mori.*

Wilfred Owen

Introduction

February 1991

I can't breathe . . .

I've put my gas mask on, twisted the canister, just like they trained us at Sandhurst, and still nothing. I desperately try to inhale again but as I try to force some air in all I can smell is baked beans on my breath, the meal I was eating on my lap just before we were attacked by Scud missiles in the darkness of the Saudi Arabian desert.

Beyond my mask I can just make out the silhouettes of my fellow soldiers all frantically racing for cover. Across from me, Squadron Sergeant Major 'Skip' Ray has slammed his mask on his face so hard he cut himself and now the mask's filling with blood. But he can breathe, and that's more than I can say.

I've been in the Gulf for three weeks. It's my first military tour, at twenty-seven years of age, and as captain attached to the 14th/20th Hussars I'm meant to know what

Introduction

I'm doing. But when someone shouts, 'GAS, GAS, GAS!' as your desert camp is unexpectedly hit in the middle of the night, serious panic sets in. And then when your gas mask doesn't work, all your training and logical thought go straight out of the window.

We all instantly think it must be sarin. After all, this is the gas we have been warned about. The scary thing about sarin is it's odourless, and colourless. You're not even sure if it's there, but before you know it there's a tightness in the chest, a constriction of the pupils, a froth on the lips. As the chemical blocks the brain's ability to control muscle movement, you go into spasm, twitching and jerking, losing control of bodily functions. Vomiting, urinating and defecating, you then slide into a coma, your heart gradually suffocated to an agonizing death. *Christ, I'd rather be shot in the head.* And that's why I can't take my mask off. I'd sooner choke to death wearing this useless mask, that is supposedly meant to protect me, than go out that way.

'Turn the valves round, you muppet!' my driver, Boo Boo Johnson, screams in my face. He's a hard-as-nails Glaswegian, who affectionately calls me 'FEB', short for 'Fucking English Bastard', but I can see in his eyes that even he is bricking it right now. 'They don't work,' I shout back, demonstrating that no matter which way I turn the valves no air is flowing. Boo Boo grips my mask and has a go himself. Nothing. My face is going redder and redder. It was red enough already after three days stuck in the searing desert so I must look like a beetroot by now.

Whoosh – Whoosh – Whoosh.

More rockets whizz past, lighting up the night sky, shaking the earth around me.

Pop-pop-pop.

Then the crackling sound of gunfire fills my ears. I'm not sure if it's them or us but suddenly the camp is alight with luminous green tracers.

Boo Boo roughly pulls my arm. 'Get down, you idiot!' he cries, as I hit the dirty floor with a thud. Just seconds before we had been sat enjoying a warm desert night, sharing stories, ripping the piss out of each other, wondering if we were ever going to see any action. Now we are right in the thick of it and I'm wondering, *What the hell am I doing here?*

The Gulf War had started just a few weeks before but had been brewing for months, ever since the Iraqi President Saddam Hussein had ordered his forces to invade neighbouring Kuwait. I must admit, I didn't know the ins and outs of it all, and I didn't particularly care. I was just a young guy who was proud to be serving his country and upholding a family tradition that had seen my grandfather and father both serve before me. I guess you could say I was an army brat, growing up in British bases all over the world. This had always been my dream, my lifelong ambition.

But if I didn't get breathing soon, it would all be over before it had really begun.

As more tracers zip overhead, Boo Boo jolts himself into combat mode and charges into the mayhem. But I stay rooted to the ground. My lungs are almost empty and my eyes pop wide, as if they're trying to drag in some air. The fizzing of bullets, yelling and explosions fill my ears but slowly the relentless cacophony becomes background noise. One by one my brain discounts them as threats. Its number one priority right now is to get some air back into the system.

What do you want me to do? my mind screams. If I keep the mask on, I'm going to choke to death. If I take it off, I'm going to be suffocated by gas. And if I stand and run, I'm going to get shot in the crossfire.

But if I don't do something, I've had it, and the first thought that comes into my head is: *I can't die. Julia will bloody kill me.*

I'd met Julia a few years before at Reading University, where I was studying agriculture, the only course I could get on to because I'd messed up my A levels. It wasn't my intention to study much anyway. I saw my three years at university as an opportunity to play some rugby and have a good time before I went off to start the serious business at the military academy at Sandhurst. Julia and I were very different in that respect. She was studying real estate management and was sensible and curious, enjoying art, museums and churches. Meanwhile, I spent my time in the Student's Union, downing pints and boorishly singing rugby songs. But as soon as I had set my eyes on her, my alpha-male ego was scrunched into a ball and thrown into the bin. Somehow, we just clicked. I knew she was the love of my life and I could never be without her. Just before I had departed for the Gulf, I had proposed. Thankfully, she'd said yes and we were due to be married on my return.

Intense anger flashes over me. *I have to survive this. I can't let Julia down.* As more screeching Scuds fly overhead, and my brigade unloads a tempest of artillery in return, I see one of our Land Rovers fifty yards away. Suddenly I know what I must do. I'm not out of the game just yet.

I steady myself. There's no time to wait for a lull in the gunfire. I'm just going to have to go at this with all I've got. It's last-chance-saloon stuff. Do or die. Adrenalin surges through me and I leap up.

Phut-phut-phut.

Ducking down, I charge forwards, somehow evading the barrage of gunfire, but the adrenalin soon wanes as the lack of oxygen hits my legs. I feel like I'm running through sludge. My heart tightens with every step. My lungs scream. My muscles burn. It's like someone is on my back, trying to force me to the ground. I look up. Everything is now a blur, sounds and colours all swirling into one. My brain is shutting down. I know if I don't make it to the Land Rover in thirty seconds the colours will soon be pitch black, and then I'm a goner.

I trip over something and stumble but I can't afford to hit the deck now, every second is precious. In the darkness I reach out, hoping to feel something, all the while closing my eyes, tipping my head back, in a desperate attempt to get another gasp of air into my lungs. And then I feel it. The Land Rover. I reach for the door handle. *Please don't be locked . . . Click!* It opens. *Thank God!*

I drag myself inside and slam the door shut. I look down. The keys are in the ignition. I turn them hard, hear the engine kick in, pull the gear stick back and slam my foot on the pedal. *VROOM!* The car careers backwards, away from the mayhem, scrunching over bits of equipment. I grip the window handle and hurriedly turn it. There's only seconds left. The window comes down and I frantically reach for my mask, praying I've left the gas behind. Slamming on the brakes, I tear off the mask and gasp for air, desperately trying to fill my lungs, and then . . .

Whoosh!

A rush of clean desert air hits me. I gulp down breath after breath. It can't have been more than a minute or two since the attack began, but it feels like I've been holding my breath for half an hour. Abruptly my vision kicks back in, and my senses return. I'm fine. I've escaped. *But I'll kill whoever fitted my valves when I find him.* And then I start to laugh. Hysterical laughter. A primal reaction to being scared.

As I look out of the window, I see my fellow soldiers just a hundred yards away, all still sporting their gas masks and fighting fire with fire. My laughter quickly turns to fear. It hits me: I almost died. The tears come first, then the shame of crying. *You're meant to be a captain in the army, for Christ's sake.* But I can't stop them now. My body needs the release. I just have to hope none of the lads see me. I'd never hear the end of it, even though I know they're all bricking it themselves.

I make a vow to myself there and then that I'll never again put myself in a situation that could involve chemical weapons. Give me a good old-fashioned gunfight any day. No amount of money will change my mind. It's funny how things turn out . . .

4 March 2018

As I came off the stage in Abu Dhabi, where I had been delivering a keynote address at a security conference, I took my phone out of my pocket and quickly gave it a glance. There were fifty-two missed calls and 108 WhatsApp messages. This was unusual. Something was clearly up.

Quickly finding a quiet corner, scanning the missed calls, I realized they were from almost every media organi-

Introduction

zation in the UK, from *The Times* to the BBC, as well as a few from America. More worryingly, I also noticed missed calls from a number I know to be from friends in the intelligence world. I decided to make them my first port of call.

Ensuring that I couldn't be heard, I dialled the number in question only to swiftly be greeted by some choice Anglo-Saxon:

'Where the hell are you?'

'I'm in Abu Dhabi,' I replied, bemused.

'We have a situation.'

I instantly assumed this must be an issue in the Middle East, most likely Syria, where I had been doing a lot of work. What came next stunned me.

'We think there has been a chemical attack in Salisbury.'

The words chilled me to my core. I lived just outside Salisbury, with Julia and our two children. I only became more concerned as my friend outlined the situation.

'Two Russians are in a serious condition. The doctors have never seen anything like it. They're frozen, like statues.'

As the seriousness of the attack dawned on me, I couldn't help but think of the irony. Though I'd vowed never to go near chemical weapons again, whenever there was a chemical attack, anywhere in the world, I was now one of the first people to get a call. In the years since the incident in the Gulf I had commanded the Chemical, Biological, Radiological and Nuclear (CBRN) Regiment, as well as NATO's CBRN Battalion. During this time, I had

Introduction

worked in war zones all over the globe, experiencing all the horrors that working in such a field can throw at you. I'd stood on the edge of mass graves in Iraq, watched in horror as children gasped their last breaths in Syria, been chased through Afghan streets while carrying a huge fertilizer bomb, joined the Kurds in facing off against ISIS, and risked my life trying to smuggle chemical samples across borders. As I write, my expertise has also been called upon to help tackle the COVID-19 outbreak.

Yet following those inauspicious beginnings in the Gulf, it seemed my career had now come full circle, as my home town of Salisbury, my supposed safe haven, had been hit. There was to be no escape. It seemed the spectre of chemical weapons had been following me all my life, no matter how hard I tried to avoid them.

Part One

'Men Marched Asleep'

1

Break-up

'I don't think we should be together any more.'

With those crushing words, Julia handed back her engagement ring. Apparently, things had been rocky since I had returned from the Gulf but I had failed to notice any of the signs.

You see, surviving an attack like the one I had been through does funny things to a person. Some go under, retreat into a shell and need counselling to process it all. That's the brave thing to do. That's how you face up to your demons and grow. Me? I ran as far away from those feelings of fear and vulnerability as possible, drowning it all in pints of beer and boys' nights out.

Did I have PTSD? It's hard to say, and back in those days there was no real talk of that type of condition anyway, so it certainly wasn't something on my radar. If you had asked me what I thought PTSD was, I probably would have told you it was a rock band. Whether more awareness would have made any difference I can't be sure. I was young and cocky, and surviving such a situation makes you feel indestructible. The initial feeling may be one of fear but once you get over that, and survive every bullet being fired in your direction, you want more. It almost becomes an addiction. The more you survive, the cockier you become. But while *I* thought I was Master of the Universe, Julia wasn't quite so enamoured. As she succinctly put it, 'You've become a bit of an arse.'

Looking back, she was right. After nine months in the Gulf, I had boarded our BA flight back home with a very high opinion of myself. Not only had I seen action but, in a lull between fighting, I had even found time to break the world press-up record, completing 4,489 in under three hours. While the *Guinness Book of Records* wasn't present to record my feat, it had been captured live on Forces Radio. In my eyes this was even better. It ensured everyone in the armed forces knew about it, from brigadiers to special forces. 'That's de Bretton-Gordon, the world press-up champ,' I would hear people whisper to their mates, as I swaggered past.

On the flight back, we were meant to be restricted to just two beers, but I felt that just wasn't going to cut it. Lashings of beer were liberally chased by shots of vodka, while my voice grew louder by the glassful. Although it must be said, I wasn't the only one who had a raging thirst. There were a fair few young officers on that flight – including my lifelong chum Dave 'Bully' Cowan, a 'bull' of a man from Cumbria – who felt they were far too important to listen to such fanciful notions as 'orders'. Thankfully, our superiors were prepared to give us a little latitude, considering none of us had touched a drop since we had set foot in the Gulf. However, I took things further than most and staggered off the plane in a very sorry state, squinting into the morning sunshine, feeling rather queasy.

For the next few months, such behaviour was par for the course. Within hours of arriving in London I had given Julia no more than a cursory peck on the cheek before I was out the front door and lapping up the nightlife in the West End. One minute I was dodging bullets and gas, the next I was downing shots in a bar and dancing to Right Said Fred.

It's no wonder my head became so messed up. There was no buffer between these two extremes. In those days, there were no decompression procedures in place, to help a soldier returning from a war zone gradually ease their way back into normality. These days, after a tour, soldiers are usually sent to a third location for a few days to wind down and become accustomed to a less intense way of life. But back then you went straight from one extreme to the other, without so much as a pause for breath. Unsurprisingly, my relationship was caught in the crossfire.

While I had been away, Julia had made a life for herself in Putney, where she was now working as a surveyor. She had a new group of friends and was mixing in very different circles to the ones I had been used to. As you might imagine, my time in the Gulf involved mixing with a group of very macho, testosterone-fuelled guys. The humour was brash and lairy, and trying to adapt to more serene surroundings, not to mention more refined company, was very difficult. I just wasn't house-trained for social niceties and found the conversations mind-numbingly boring, something I wasn't afraid to express by constantly yawning and checking the time whenever we did go out.

Julia always reminds me of one particular incident during a welcome-home dinner party at my parents' house. During a news report we were watching on soldiers return-ing from the Gulf, a reporter asked one of them, 'What are you looking forward to the most?' to which the young comedian dryly remarked, 'Shagging.' At this I declared, in front of my parents and guests, 'If anyone deserves any shagging, it's me!' My family were from military circles, so such displays of bravado were somewhat expected from a young idiot back from his first tour, but for Julia it was understandably mortifying.

Not only did I find it hard to adapt to her new life but I also didn't want to discuss my time in the Gulf with her. If I actually opened up about what really happened out there, I felt that my war-hero status would come under question and my macho façade might crumble. You see, despite appearances, I was harbouring a deep shame. It had turned out that my apparent brush with chemical weapons was a

16

false alarm. Soon after the attack, we found there was no sarin in the rockets, and at no point did Saddam deploy chemical weapons during the Gulf War. He certainly had them, but he knew that if he set them loose then he would have been facing Armageddon. But despite this, I had felt the fear. I had truly believed I was under attack by sarin and I had been unable to breathe due to my defective gas mask. Psychologically, that was enough. I had been genuinely terrified, as if it was the real thing. So, while everyone was treating me like a hero, deep down I was too embarrassed to tell them it had been a false alarm. Sure, I had seen some action, but in my mind heroes don't confess that they were terrified by a false alarm, so much so that it moved them to tears and continued to plague them.

More than that, I didn't actually want to talk about any of it. The anxiety of going off to war. The fear of being in a gunfight. The long days just waiting for something to happen. I didn't even want to talk about the moments of excitement. It seemed to me that if I just kept my mouth shut then people would continue to believe I was a war hero.

But it wasn't just war that had made me this way. This was a by-product of my childhood, which had taught me that military men don't talk about their feelings. From the moment I was born, the military was ingrained into me. My father, Alistair, had been with the Royal Signals for over forty years and had seen action in the Korean War.

His brothers had done likewise, all of them rising to the rank of colonel. Not once can I remember any of them talking about their emotions. They were very old-fashioned in that respect. We didn't hug, we shook hands. If I were to fall and cut my knee, my father would scold, 'Sons of army officers don't cry.'

As my parents were stationed abroad, I was sent to boarding school when I was six. Again, this was not an environment where showing emotion was permitted. If you so much as shed a tear, you could expect to be picked on for the rest of your schooldays, and that was just by the teachers! The real test for all of us boarders was how you would react to being caned. I've lost count of the number of times I received this particular brand of punishment, for a litany of misdemeanours. I was a happy but cheeky child, full of energy and mischief and sometimes that over-exuberance got me into trouble. It was never anything too serious, but when talking after lights out was treated as a major crime, you can imagine what would happen if you were caught smoking out of the windows. In my time I would pay the price for both of these dreadful crimes, as well as a few others.

Punishment was usually dished out just before supper, so after 'six of the best' you then had to endure the walk of shame into the dining hall. Everyone would turn as you entered, limping gingerly to your seat, the whole hall full of eyes burning into you. How would you take the beating?

Would you stand tall like a man? Or would you limp to your seat with tears streaming down your cheeks?

I remember as an eight-year-old walking past the 'big kids' with my backside throbbing, while they all eyed me up like hungry prey, willing me to crack. *Don't look at them, Hamish,* I told myself. *You'll never live it down.* To show any emotion whatsoever would have led to me being ostracized for months. To stop my eyes from moistening, I bit my lip so hard that I pierced the skin and could taste blood in my mouth. Somehow, to the dining hall's intense disappointment, I made it to my seat without my façade crumbling, but such was the deep bruising that I had to squat on the loo for weeks.

However, this walk along the green mile soon became a badge of honour. As a teenager I almost relished the chance to swagger into that hall after being caned, to show just how big and tough I was. 'Easy,' I'd say to my friends with a wink, as I gingerly sat my bruised backside down to eat. In fact, after the trials and tribulations of boarding school, I actually found Sandhurst Military Academy a breeze. 'Two hundred press-ups, sir? Not a problem!' All done with a smile on my face, no grumbling at all. I even rather enjoyed it.

So, as you can imagine, after all of this, showing emotion was not something that came naturally to me. Yet I must say that I had a very happy childhood. This is certainly not a memoir of a tough upbringing by emotionally distant parents that sent me off the rails, desperate for a hug. Quite the opposite, in fact. I was a normal, happy-go-lucky kid who faced no real hardships in life. Unlike others, I actually loved school. I was always in the thick of it with my mates, and played sport as often as I could, excelling in rugby and cricket. By and large, the teachers were great, and while my relationship with my parents was old-fashioned, I always felt very loved. We all got on together very well, and continue to do so.

However, there's no getting away from the fact that my military upbringing, coupled with boarding school, trained me to always act like the cocky guy who wasn't worried about anything. On the surface I was rock steady. Nothing seemed to bother me at all. Every situation was met with a laugh and a joke, my self-defence mechanism immediately kicking in.

Yet after my experiences in the Gulf, while on the surface I seemed on top of the world, deep down I was suffering. Since the attack, my nightmares had become increasingly vivid. Clouds of gas would envelop me in the darkness, as a dark void swallowed me whole, leaving me choking for air. I would wake with a start, soaked in sweat, struggling to breathe, panting and wheezing, just as I had been in the desert. Yet now I had Julia sleeping next to me, which was a tremendous comfort. In the darkness I would reach for her hand and squeeze it tight. I would then lie there for hours, the supposed hero, eyes open wide, just staring at the ceiling, too afraid to go back to sleep, counting the seconds until sunrise.

As I said, any talk of my experiences in the Gulf with Julia was a no-go zone. Any attempt she made to bring it up was immediately shot down. If I felt she was prying, or complaining about my emotionally vacant state, I'd change the subject or fly off the handle. Anything to keep her at arm's length. To avoid any of this, all I wanted was to go out night after night, with guys who had shared experiences similar to mine, and get totally obliterated. If that wasn't a sign that perhaps all was not well, then there were other things lurking just below the surface.

I had always been a very keen rugby player and swiftly laced up my boots on my return. However, this time my mentality was different. While I had always been a very aggressive player, now I was really taking things to the edge. Not only were some of my tackles high and dangerous but I also found myself becoming embroiled in fist fights. It was almost as if I saw a rugby match as a legitimate place to unleash my underlying fury at being so scared in the Gulf. I even earned the nickname DLT – Deliberate Late Tackle. And this mentality sometimes spilled over into nights out, where at any sign of trouble I was usually the first to throw a punch. Deep down I knew this wasn't me, that I was acting out against all of my fears, but I had no idea how to handle it.

Unsurprisingly, it didn't take Julia too long to tire of her regularly drunk, black-eyed lout of a fiancé. Attractive, funny, kind and successful, Julia had no reason to put up with such behaviour. She had spent all the time that I was away worried sick about me. Now I was back, I was behaving as if I couldn't care less. Soon she reached breaking point. Having organized an afternoon boating on the river in Richmond, she had no doubt hoped for a romantic few hours together. To her, this was a chance for us to be totally alone, where she hoped that I might relax, open up, or even just sit back and feel at peace in the London sunshine for the first time since I had been home. Sadly, I didn't take the bait. Instead I moaned about how bored I was and fired off a series of lewd jokes. Finally, she snapped. 'Hamish, for Christ's sake, just shut up!' It was the first time someone had managed to get me to shut my mouth in weeks.

Yet even as Julia proceeded to tell me what an arrogant bore I had become and handed her engagement ring back to me, I struggled to feel remorse for my actions. I'm ashamed to think of it now, but at the time I still felt she was lucky to have me and not the other way around. This was a line I would drunkenly tell my friends over and over, while I continued to prop up the bar for the next few weeks. I refused to admit that *I* might be the problem, which I can now see, with years of hindsight, and hopefully maturity, that I clearly was. It's a funny thing but when you get older you cringe at some of the things you've done in your life. This period is definitely one of them. But as the weeks went by, and more of my drinking buddies settled down and returned to normality, soon there was no one left to go out with. I was all alone.

Back living at my parents' flat in Notting Hill Gate, I eventually had no choice but to reflect on what had happened and who I had become. In the darkness of the quiet nights the events of the Gulf would continue to wake me up in a cold sweat. And now there was no one next to me. Even if I might not have talked to Julia about the Gulf, I now realized just what a comforting presence she had been.

I began to miss her terribly. From her ebullient, can-do attitude to the smell of the Cacharel Anaïs Anaïs lemon perfume that she always wore. I even missed her somewhat bossy attitude. While I might have complained about it, she always seemed to know best and had kept me grounded. Without her, I was lost at sea, swamped in solitude and the chaos of my own head. I soon realized just what 'an arse' I had become. If I didn't do something soon, I would mess up the most important thing in my life.

But despite all that, I still couldn't pick up the phone. To do so would be to publicly admit that I was wrong. And while I already knew that, it was another step altogether to admit such a thing to Julia. Male pride can be a terrible thing. Yet those dark nights alone didn't get any easier, and soon the thought of all those eligible young bachelors nipping at Julia's heels tipped me over the edge.

Finally, I made the call. Trying to play it cool, I nonchalantly said I was just checking in to see how she was doing. Most importantly, I did my best to avoid acting like a moron, which was very hard indeed. For her part, Julia didn't make it easy on me. I had hoped she would come rushing back, greeting me with her arms wide open, but I was still very much in the deep freeze. This only spurred me on to make greater efforts. Soon I was forgoing booze and back in the gym, trying to get back to my old self, while bombarding her with flowers, chocolates and anything else I could think of in the name of romance.

Thankfully, it did the trick. After weeks of me proving that I was really trying my best, Julia gradually warmed to my overtures. Soon the engagement was back on and in September 1992 we were married, at Woburn Abbey. I was a very happy and very lucky man. I knew how close I had come to losing her. I felt re-energized with her alongside me, more settled within myself. Everything appeared to be coming up roses. But as I would find out time and time again in my career, the world of chemical weapons, and war, was never far away.

2

New Assignment

'Tough break, DBG.'

To me, the news I had just received from the Colonel Commandant of the Royal Tank Regiment (RTR) was the ultimate insult. My colleagues' sympathetic glances, shaking of their heads and pats on the back showed they also felt I had received a raw deal.

With over a decade as an officer in the RTR behind me, and with war erupting in Iraq, I was expecting to be promoted to command my own regiment. It was 2004, I was forty-one years of age and I had risen through all the required ranks, earning combat experience in the Gulf along the way. All of the reports I had received had been complimentary, and I had passed all of my exams with flying colours. I'd waited my whole life for this moment and had made my fair share of sacrifices for it. Now I was being told it was not to be. Rather than command an RTR regiment I would instead be in charge of something rather more obscure: the Chemical, Biological, Radiological and Nuclear (CBRN) Regiment.

In 1999, the Royal Tank Regiment had taken over command of the CBRN Regiment, for no real reason other than a typical military fudge to save money (the Territorials had previously fulfilled this function on a part-time basis). However, I must admit the creation of a full-time CBRN regiment had somewhat passed me by. Following my experience in the Gulf, I had shown no inclination whatsoever to be involved with chemical weapons. I was more than happy in my tank, thank you very much.

Yet for some mysterious reason, my superiors had now decided that I was just the man for the vacant CBRN role. I have no idea why this was the case. I had no scientific background whatsoever. In fact, I was terrible at science in school. While I had studied combined sciences at O level, which to put it kindly was for students with no academic ability, I had crashed out of biology at A level, and had then achieved only a third-class degree in agriculture. I was hardly the next Einstein.

I had also shown that I was absolutely terrified of a gas attack. I wanted no part of chemical warfare. Fourteen years on from the Gulf and the flashbacks and nightmares still had the ability to wake me up in a cold sweat. Now I would be in command of a regiment that was supposed to deal with such attacks on a regular basis. It felt like I was being consigned to hell.

And it wasn't as if I had shown an interest in this subject since the Gulf, in an effort to understand chemical weapons and try to face my demons. Far from it. I had actually done all I could to avoid the subject at all costs. If there was ever anything in the news about chemical weapons, I would change the channel. I operated on an out of sight, out of mind basis. The more I thought about it all the more it made no sense. What the hell did I know about chemical weapons to be in such a position of authority? All I knew was how to run away from them! This was not how I had envisioned my career panning out. Commanding a tank regiment had always been my dream. Anything to do with chemical weapons was a total nightmare.

Tanks had captured my imagination since the age of six. I can still vividly recall sitting on my dad's shoulders at a British military parade in Bahrain, amongst thousands of others, watching soldiers march to the beat of a military band. I was entranced. Rifles were being fired into the air, huge jeeps and rocket launchers were trundling past, while swords and various guns all caught my eager eye. But then the sun bounced off a hunk of gleaming metal, momentarily blinding me. As I squinted to get a better look, my vision suddenly came back into focus and then my whole world was turned upside down.

Before me was a giant green monster, with the biggest gun I'd ever seen. 'What's that, Dad?' I asked, in awe. 'It's a

Centurion tank,' he answered. *A Centurion tank . . .* I said the words under my breath again and again, as if I knew I had to remember this, that this was somehow going to play a major part of my life. That one day it was going to be me inside that monster, and then my life would be complete. It's a memory that has never left me.

Whenever I see the movie *Goodfellas* I always smile at the immortal Ray Liotta line: 'For as long as I can remember, I wanted to be a gangster.' For me, it's: 'For as long as I can remember, I wanted to be a Tankie.' That was all I ever wanted in life. Perhaps this is the reason I did so poorly at school, gaining very mediocre grades at A level. I wasn't concerned in the slightest: I had already earmarked my future, and it was to command a tank in a war zone.

I was certainly in the right environment to encourage this ambition. Every school holiday I was whisked off to whichever military base my parents were stationed at. I loved military bases. They were my Disneyland as a child. There was always a gang of kids looking for something to do, and we had no shortage of options. There were tennis and basketball courts, football and rugby pitches, not to mention lots of places to get up to mischief. I'd spend all summer in the sunshine, playing sport. But more than sport, more than anything in fact, what really got my blood pumping was already feeling like I was a part of the military, like I was doing an apprenticeship. What child, with the opportunity to watch soldiers at close quarters, wouldn't get a buzz from it all? And every so often those tanks would roll on to a base and totally captivate me.

I became obsessed with them. There was a time I could tell you anything you wanted to know, from the track size of a Chieftain to the size of a gun on a Challenger I. If I wasn't drawing them, I would be trying to touch them or, better yet, speak to someone who had actually driven one. The biggest thrill of all was that my dad's friend, Brigadier Nick Cocking, was actually in the Royal Tank Regiment. He might as well have been in the Rolling Stones. Every chance I got I pumped him for information: 'What does it look like inside?' 'How do you fire the gun?' 'How do you drive it?' Nick very kindly indulged my passion and in turn took me under his wing, not only answering my many questions but also giving me various insignia, which I proudly displayed on my wall, alongside posters of Gareth Edwards and Ian Botham. Those idols were soon consigned to the bin as I learnt about the courageous feats of General Montgomery, who against all odds had led the British to victory over the Germans in the Battle of El Alamein in the Second World War. Incidentally, my grandfather also served at El Alamein, as the regimental doctor of one of the infantry battalions, which only increased my interest even more.

In the early 80s, as I became a teenager, it seemed I was far from the only one who thought that being in the military was the cool thing to do. I remember a call coming out from the dining room of my boarding school in 1980: 'They're going in! Look at this!' At this we all ran to the small black-and-white television, fitted high in the corner of the room. On it we saw flickering images of SAS soldiers, sporting black balaclavas, tossing smoke bombs into the Iranian Embassy in London. Soon after, they emerged triumphant, having rescued nineteen hostages from the clutches of terrorists. It looked like something out of a movie. We watched in silence as these live pictures were broadcast around the world, making the SAS into rock stars. Their names still roll off the tongue now: John McAleese . . . Tom MacDonald . . . Rusty Firmin. It still gives me goosebumps just thinking about it. *Bloody hell!* It was fantastic!

Two years later, the British military was again being exalted high and wide as the Falklands War with the Argentines erupted. For hours I would watch the news or read the newspapers, transfixed, particularly as a school friend was over there fighting. James Stewart had been two years above me but had left school as soon as he could to attend Sandhurst. At just nineteen, he now found himself commanding a Scots Guard platoon during the Battle of Mount Tumbledown. I found it amazing that a few months before we had been smoking behind a bike shed together and now he was in the heart of battle. A real soldier. A real man.

All of the teachers and pupils used to stop to watch any news from the Falklands to see if we could spot James. He was a hero to all of us and remains a great friend to this day. I was so jealous. It all looked so exciting. As soon as I got a chance I wanted to follow in his footsteps, flying out to far-flung exotic hotspots, fighting alongside my mates, and then coming home to get a medal pinned on my chest in front of an adoring crowd. And all in the name of Queen and country. To me, that seemed like heaven.

I had no time for academic work and had no interest in any other career. The thought of a life behind a desk appalled me. All I wanted from life was to join the army, sit in a tank and be a hero. The ins and outs of war didn't concern me in the slightest. I would have fought anywhere, at any time. Just let me at them!

When, after university, I was commissioned into the 4th Royal Tank Regiment (4 RTR), I was elated. It felt as though I was going to play for Manchester United. Finally, I would have the thrill of being inside those tremendous monsters and hopefully one day follow in the footsteps of the likes of General Montgomery. But there was a snag. The regiment's barracks were based in Germany, which gave Julia and I, the newly married couple, quite a dilemma. She had a well-paid, secure job in London. Her life was there, and she had worked tremendously hard to build up her career. But she also knew that this was my dream. Making a huge sacrifice, she offered to come with me to Germany. Words can't express my gratitude. I knew how much she was giving up, not to mention that she wouldn't know a soul out there and also didn't know the language. But Julia being Julia, she immediately got stuck in, and had soon acquired a job on the military newspaper, which she rather enjoyed.

As for me, I was truly living out all of my dreams. Finally being able to clamber inside a Chieftain tank and fire that gun was really something. For those initial few months, I must have fired more ammo than anyone in the British Army. I couldn't get enough of it. I was like a big kid.

We'd usually have exercises where old tank hulks were set out as targets two miles away. I'd absolutely hammer them! Feeling the power of the gun recoil, then the booming sound as it sent a projectile hurtling at 1,500 metres per second to explode the target was an unbelievable rush. Back home, people my age were losing their minds to acid house. Well, my rave was inside a tank, blasting the crap out of things. Of course, this was all fun and games. As if I was playing with my mates in the playground, with no danger of any harm coming to anyone. The reality of such monsters on the battlefield is very different. They are truly killing machines and it is quite shocking to see the damage they can do in reality.

From troop leader I was soon promoted to squadron leader, and I was also set loose in Challenger 1 and Challenger 2 tanks, the Premier League of tanks. Now all I wanted was a chance to blow the enemy away in a war zone. Chance would have been a fine thing.

By the mid 90s the world seemed to be in a settled state. The Gulf War was won and the Cold War, which had plagued the world for decades, had also come to an end following the collapse of the Soviet Union. And while issues in Northern Ireland rumbled on, the situation there was nowhere near as intense as it had once been. In any event, 4 RTR wasn't deployed in the province.

With no conflicts on the horizon, all there was to do was train. Hour after hour, day after day, week after week. Soon even firing the gun at targets started to wear thin. I craved the real thing but, apart from a brief tour of Bosnia and Croatia in 1995, it seemed as though I was destined for a succession of training exercises.

I found this incredibly frustrating. I longed to see some action. That was why I had joined the military, not for endless exercises and courses. I dreamt of commanding the tank regiment in the heat of war, where this time I wouldn't be running from gas but charging head first into battle, protected by a steel shell and a booming arsenal. Deep down, I still felt some shame from what had happened in the Gulf, and I longed for a chance to prove myself on the battlefield.

While there were no wars on the horizon, another very welcome opportunity soon presented itself. Anyone who has any aspirations to progress in the army must complete the Army Command and Staff College. This focuses on the things that all prospective commanders must grasp, such as staff and communication skills, as well as command leadership and management. However, competition for places is intense. Only 25% of applicants make it and for those who don't, it's pretty much a career death sentence. The highest rank anyone could realistically expect to achieve without passing this course is lieutenant colonel. There are many who leave the military altogether if they fail to get a place, their dreams scuppered. To my great surprise, I was one of the chosen few. And while I could opt to take the course back in the UK, there was a far more alluring option for Julia and me: Australia.

This was a tremendous experience for a young married couple. It certainly didn't take us long to take to the sunshine and the Australian way of life. Settling in Melbourne, we learnt to surf, ate well and revelled in the more laidback lifestyle. I even managed to play semi-professional Aussie Rules football, although I think they just enjoyed having a token 'Pom' on the team to take the piss out of, something I had no problem with, as I was happy giving it back in spades. Whenever I would run out in front of a couple of hundred people, I'd hear, 'There he is! There's the Pom!' At this I'd blow them kisses, which always wound them up.

Despite all the fun, there was still a lot of hard work to get through, and at times I still had to spend days or weeks away from Julia. But as usual, she was never short of friends and travelled all over that beautiful country. We also enjoyed many trips together and had a tremendous time. I came to love this way of life. Swimming in the surf, with the sun beating down on us both, I remember thinking: *This'll do me.*

Sadly, our time in paradise was soon at an end. Within twelve months I had passed the course and we had to return to Germany. Neither of us were enthused by this prospect but we soon had exciting news to lift our spirits: Julia was pregnant with our daughter, Jemima. This was a real thrill for us both.

Jemima was born on 15 June 1997 in a German hospital, where I discovered that it was customary for the fathers to look after the baby in a crèche for the first twelve hours while the mother slept and recovered. I was terrified as a nurse handed this tiny little person to me and told me to bathe and feed her. I didn't have a clue what to do. The sense of responsibility was almost overwhelming, but having that initial time together really allowed me to feel a strong bond with her. I didn't want to leave her side and would watch over her as she slept, constantly checking if she was still breathing. I was well and truly infatuated.

Sadly, after just a few days with Julia and Jemima in Germany, I was sent to Canada for three months, for more training exercises, and then on to Cyprus, for a six-month operational United Nations' tour. In Jemima's first year, I was home for only nineteen days, which was agonizing. I hated being away from her and Julia, and back in those days, before the widespread use of mobile phones and the internet, we were only given a phone card which gave me thirty minutes of calls a week. More often than not we had to resort to writing letters. But hearing that I had missed out on seeing Jemima's first steps or hearing her first words hurt me terribly.

I also began to feel tremendously guilty. Julia was shouldering all of the burden, running herself into the ground. By now she had been abroad with me for six years and had already sacrificed so much. Having to continually leave her to single-handedly look after a baby who viewed sleeping as anathema was awful. Julia didn't complain (much) but I could tell it was getting her down. And it wasn't as if I was off saving the world, so could justify my jaunts to myself. It was just yet more training exercises, and climbing the ranks. In the circumstances, it was clear what I had to do. As such, in 1999, I requested a transfer home and was sent to Salisbury, where I was consigned to a desk job, planning training exercises of all things!

At least being at home allowed my guilt to somewhat subside, and I could enjoy more time watching Jemima grow up. And as Julia was now surrounded by friends and family, and resuming her career as a surveyor, she was much happier, especially when a year later we welcomed our son, Felix, into the world. Yet I now felt adrift. I was rising through the ranks quickly, now a lieutenant colonel, but I spent most of my days sitting behind a desk, the last thing I had ever wanted. Where was the action? Where was the thrill? My father had served for forty years in the military and had only ever seen action in Korea. Was this to also be my fate? Would my experience in the Gulf prove to be it?

One September afternoon, as I settled down for some lunch, I turned on the TV to see a breaking news story flash on to the screen. Two planes had crashed into the Twin Towers in New York. As the details became clearer, my immediate thoughts were with my cousin and his wife. They both worked as bankers in one of the towers. The next few hours were fraught. Desperately, I tried to find out if they were safe, while I watched in horror as the towers both fell, and further planes crashed into the Pentagon and a field in Pennsylvania. Thankfully, news soon reached me that they had escaped the towers before they collapsed, but with that relief came the dawning realization that the world had irrevocably changed. War was back on the horizon, first in Afghanistan, and then in Iraq.

It seemed my time had come. Finally, I might get the chance to command a tank regiment in a war zone. Yet it was not to be; my dreams came to a crushing end the moment the Colonel Commandant delivered the news that I was to instead command the CBRN Regiment.

I was distraught. Commanding a tank regiment was seen by many to be where the real action was, where heroes were forged and legends were made. It was also perceived by most that to reach the highest ranks in the armed forces you had to have commanded a guards, cavalry or rifles regiment. The CBRN Regiment was none of these. I felt as if I was effectively being demoted. For over a decade I had toiled, without a war zone in sight, and now we were at war my dream had been snatched away from me. It was as if they were saying, 'You're not made of the right stuff, DBG. Leave the real army to us.'

I was livid, and expected Julia to share my disappointment. After all, she had made tremendous sacrifices, all so that I could one day command an RTR. Now it all appeared to have been for nothing. Yet as I relayed my anger, she was strangely calm. 'Don't you see, Hamish? This is a huge opportunity for you!' I began to calm down as I realized that, as usual, she might be right.

Despite my love for the RTR, it was evident that tank warfare was dying out. War had become less conventional and far more complex, with tanks now rarely deployed on the battlefield. These days, most conflicts seem to be dealt with by aircraft, spies or special forces operations, as seen in the 2001 invasion of Afghanistan, where a small team of special forces, aided by bomber aircraft, took control of the whole country. The days of armies actually facing each other head to head on the ground seemed to be a thing of the past.

Slowly but surely I came around to the idea that maybe CBRN fitted into modern warfare better than the RTR. In time, this would be where the action was, particularly with so much talk of weapons of mass destruction in Iraq, on which more later.

Indeed, the CBRN Regiment was hardly insignificant, boasting over 450 men and women amongst its ranks. And as it was still relatively new, I also thought it would really allow me to make my mark. But when it all came down to it, I didn't have much choice in the matter. These were my orders and I had to follow them. I also had a young family I needed to support, so I was certainly in no position to turn down a perceived promotion, no matter my personal feelings on the matter. As such, I had to salute, turn to the right and carry on.

'Are you looking forward to your command, DBG?'

'Can't wait to get started, sir!'

But deep down inside, owing to my previous experience in the Gulf, I was afraid. I would be heading back to the scene of my greatest fear, not in a heavily protected tank but commanding a regiment actively looking for weapons of mass destruction. Before I could take on such a tremendous responsibility, I had to get my act together, and fast.

3

The First Step

There was no getting away from it. I would be commanding the CBRN Regiment in Iraq. But I knew next to nothing on the subject, so I would have to retrain. But it would require a hell of a lot of work to get me up to speed before I was packed off to one of the most volatile war zones the world had ever seen.

With this in mind, I was sent to the Royal Military College of Science in Shrivenham to complete a chem bio science diploma. I think I was actually dreading doing the course more than facing gas on the battlefield. As I said, I had been useless in school and was terrified of showing myself up in a classroom. Military types are not the most forgiving if you should ask a foolish question and, trust me, I had plenty of them to ask. At this stage, much of what I knew about chemical weapons came from movies like *The Rock*, and I wasn't entirely sure how much of that was fact or fiction.

However, as I took my seat, along with twenty-five other supposedly eager students, and the lecture began, a strange feeling came over me. This was actually really rather interesting. Rather than doodling on the pad of paper in front of me, as the person to my right was doing, I found myself transfixed by what was being said.

I had assumed that the use of chemicals on the battle-field had been a twentieth-century development but it turned out that primitive forms of chemical and biological warfare had been around for thousands of years. As far back as 429 BC, during the siege of Plataea, Spartan soldiers built a substantial woodpile outside the city wall. When this was ignited, toxic sulphur dioxide gas was released over the walls, poisoning the defenders and forcing the Plataeans to abandon their posts. At this, the victorious Spartans strolled into Plataea and claimed their prize. In other conflicts, wells were deliberately poisoned with the bodies of dead soldiers, plants and/or animals, in order to spread disease and so cripple the enemy. Using chemicals, and disease too, in this manner soon became popular ways to break sieges when physical force would not suffice.

Another early example of a similar attack occurred in what is modern-day Syria. Archaeologists found evidence that in 256 AD twenty Roman soldiers barricaded them-selves into a tunnel, in Dura-Europos, an ancient Roman city. As a siege endured, and with the soldiers apparently safe, their enemies filled the tunnel with the fumes of burning sulphur crystals and bitumen. After inhaling this poisonous gas, all of the soldiers were soon dead.

The Tartar army in the fourteenth century perhaps conjured up the craziest attack of all. In order to capture the Crimean town of Kaffa, the Tartars catapulted the bodies of plague victims over the walls, taking the city when its inhabitants had all fallen ill. This attack seems to have inspired the Russians, who used similar techniques against the Swedes in the eighteenth century. The British also got in on the act, trying to wipe out the Native Americans by providing them with blankets that had been deliberately infected with smallpox.

However, the accidental discovery of chlorine in 1774 took chemical warfare to another level. A pulmonary agent, chlorine gas kills or incapacitates by destroying the lining of the lungs, causing them to fill with fluid and preventing them from being able to absorb oxygen, steadily choking the victim to death. During the American Civil War, both sides considered the use of chlorine as a weapon, a sign that this deadly gas could soon wreak havoc on the battlefield. Such was the concern over this that the Hague Convention attempted to ban its use in 1899. Yet chlorine gas would soon come to define modern warfare.

As the First World War exploded in 1914, the conflict between the German and Allied forces quickly descended into trench warfare. Launching wave after wave of infantry attacks, each of the two sides subsequently sought in vain to push the other back from their position. Over the coming months, hundreds of thousands perished in these attempts, with hardly any ground gained. There seemed no way to break the deadlock, other than to repeat the same horrifying pattern, again and again.

Then, on 22 April 1915, the Germans suddenly put down their guns and instead opened the valves of 6,000 cylinders of liquid chlorine. As the poisonous gas hissed from the cylinders, and came into contact with the air, it vaporized to form a five-foot-high greenish-yellow cloud. Catching the breeze, it steadily rolled across no-man's land, making its way towards the Allied trenches. The soldiers on lookout weren't particularly alarmed by this. None of them had ever seen chemical weapons in action before, so they had no idea what was coming. Therefore, as the cloud approached, there was not yet any panic. That was soon to change.

As the cloud enveloped tens of thousands of troops, their throats became inflamed, producing fluid which blocked their windpipes and filled their lungs. Gasping for breath, and frothing at the mouth, soldier after soldier quickly dropped dead. As I think back to my own experience in the Gulf, I can't imagine the sheer terror and panic these poor souls must have felt, being the first to come under attack from such a weapon, without any protection and not knowing what was happening. It is no wonder that survivors continued to be tormented by the experience for decades to come.

With the chlorine having taken effect, the Germans now emerged. Wearing moist gauze and cotton tied around their faces, acting as crude respirators, they marched, unchallenged, towards the Allied trenches. Before them was an unprecedented scene of horror. The dead lay where they had fallen, while the wounded and dying coughed up yellow fluid so violently that some ruptured their lungs. The devastating effect on the human body was clear to see, as was the gas's effect on metal. Buttons, watches and coins had all turned a dull green, while rifles that minutes before had been gleaming were now riddled with rust, looking as if they had been left out in the mud for months.

In a matter of hours the Germans had smashed defences that had held for months. Over 5,000 were dead and 10,000 wounded. From this point there would be no return. In the most horrific of circumstances, gas warfare had truly proven its worth.

With no time to waste, a chemical arms race quickly developed. This saw the British open their chemical warfare establishment at Porton Down, a 7,000 acre site on Salisbury Plain, where over 1,000 scientists were employed to create the next wave of chemical weapons.

So began three long years of chemical warfare, with ever deadlier forms of attack being utilized. First the British retaliated with phosgene, which was eighteen times more powerful than chlorine. However, unlike chlorine, phosgene was colourless and odourless, and also caused a delayed reaction, making it far more difficult to detect. After its first use at the Somme in June 1916, soldiers who innocently inhaled the gas did not realize they had done so until forty-eight hours later when they felt as if they were being drowned from within, coughing up pint after pint of yellow liquid.

In retaliation the Germans developed a so-called vesicant agent, known as mustard gas. A brown liquid that gave off a smell unsurprisingly said to be 'mustard-like', it could work its way through layers of material to attack the skin, rather than needing to be inhaled. On contact, this caused terrible pus-filled blisters to erupt, while the victims would continuously vomit, and scratch at their eyes, feeling as though sand had been thrown into them. Gradually, their windpipes were clogged from top to bottom, causing a slow and agonizing death.

While mustard gas was deadly, it also had another advantage over the likes of chlorine and phosgene. Due to its exceptional persistence, it could contaminate areas long after it had been used. Chlorine would quickly evaporate but mustard gas would form liquid pools in shell craters, ready to trap the unwary. In cold weather it also froze like water. Mustard gas that had been used in the winter of 1917 thawed in the spring of 1918, still highly dangerous and difficult to detect. In this way, mustard gas was used to seal off whole areas of a battlefield. In order to survive such conditions, men had to wear masks, leggings, gloves and googles, a huge inconvenience, which was said to reduce their efficiency on the battlefield by as much as 25%.

At this point our lecturer used a phrase I will never forget: 'As you can see, these are morbidly brilliant weapons.' 'Brilliant' was hardly the word that came to mind at that moment, but he was right. From gas there is no escape. It can be released from out of harm's way, spreading like an invisible secret agent, slipping into nooks and crannies, maiming and murdering anyone in its path, even if they try to hide. As effective weapons, they certainly are 'brilliant', but they're also downright evil. They kill indiscriminately, suffocating non-combatants who have no protection or even any warning that they are under attack.

In 1918, a twenty-nine-year-old corporal called Adolf Hitler was amongst those who was temporarily blinded by mustard gas during an attack by the British. Such was the distress of the future Führer that it has been claimed that this was among the many reasons why he did not deploy chemical weapons on the battlefield during the Second World War. Yet the Nazis did, of course, commit even worse crimes than this in secret, by gassing millions of Jews during the Holocaust, the most cowardly and diabolical act of genocide that mankind has ever seen.

By the end of the First World War gas had inflicted more than one million casualties and killed an estimated 91,000. Poems, such as 'Dulce et Decorum Est', written by Wilfred Owen in 1917 (seen at the start of this book), emphatically outlined the revulsion felt by most at the use of such weapons. An anti-gas movement subsequently grew, resulting in the 1925 Geneva Protocol, which prohibited the use of chemical weapons and outlined severe repercussions for non-compliance. However, the Protocol did not prohibit the development, production or stockpiling of such weapons. Many countries therefore continued to develop them for a few more decades, including the British at Porton Down, in the process creating the most terrifying weapons the world has ever known, as I was soon to find out.

As there was no area big enough in Britain, or indeed Europe for that matter, to allow the British Army to undertake large-scale chemical warfare exercises, we were packed off to the British Army Training Unit at Suffield (BATUS) in Alberta, Canada. This place was massive – about a fifth of the area of Northern Ireland. Its sheer size allowed the British Army to conduct exercises that UK military bases simply couldn't accommodate, such as simulating a terrorist chemical attack. For specialist troops and civil response agencies, this kind of training was critical. It helped us to fully prepare for what we might encounter on the battle-field or in a terrorism scenario, by developing what we called 'Tactics, Techniques and Procedures' (TTPs) under the world's most stringent and rigorous safety regime. Incidents in recent years, such as in Salisbury, have proved their worth.

Meanwhile, in the classroom, we learnt that sarin had been invented by the Nazis in 1936 and that the Germans had had huge stockpiles of the chemical, but due in part to Hitler's aversion to deploying chemical weapons, he never used them. However, as I was shortly due to head to Iraq, I was slightly unnerved to hear that Saddam Hussein held the honour of being the first leader to use sarin, as well as many other chemical agents, during the war with Iran in the 1980s. According to the US State Department, over 20,000 Iranian soldiers were killed by Iraqi chemical attacks during this conflict. Perhaps even more disturbing was the fact that Saddam even used nerve agents against his own people: in 1988, the Iraqi Air Force dropped 100 litre canister bombs containing a cocktail of agents, including sarin, on to the Kurdish village of Halabja, killing thousands of civilians in the process.

Yet while we kept sarin at arm's length in Canada, I would soon be working with other, more deadly nerve agents that Saddam had also a proven liking for. In an open fume cupboard, I manipulated a mixture that was the viscosity and colour of light honey. It didn't look dangerous at all, and I felt quite confident as I stirred it with a glass rod.

'In your hands you are holding the nerve agent VX,' a scientist told us. 'It is 50,000 times more potent than chlorine and many times more potent than sarin.'

Ever the smart arse, I asked the scientist how deadly were the few centimetres I held in my hand.

'If you were to correctly distribute what you are holding,' he warned, 'then you could kill one million people.'

I quickly put the mixture down, my hands shaking somewhat. How could such a small amount of mixture kill so many people? It made the mind boggle and made me realize just why dictators like Saddam craved such weapons.

British scientists had accidentally invented VX in 1952, when trying to develop a new pesticide. However, its discovery soon came to highlight a change in direction for Porton Down. In the past, the British had actively sought to develop chemical and biological weapons, such as VX, to be used on the battlefield, but by 1956 it had decided to renounce them. Humanitarian reasons played a part in this decision, although it was also due to the fragile post-war British economy and the fact that such weapons had played no part in the Second World War. All remaining stocks of chemical and biological weapons were subsequently sent to the bottom of the sea, just off the Inner Hebrides, while all research on new nerve gas weapons was cancelled. From here on, although Porton Down still researched chemical and biological weapons, it no longer manufactured them. Its focus became more defence minded. Many NATO countries also abandoned their stockpiles around this time, as it became increasingly clear to Western nations that use of such weapons was unacceptable. Thereafter, only small, specialist research facilities such as the Defence Science and Technology Laboratory (DstL) were kept on to ensure the scientific base understood the science of the weapons and how enemies might develop and use them.

While Porton Down continues its research into chemical and biological weapons, even manufacturing small samples for research purposes, today it also plays a leading role in researching deadly diseases, such as Ebola and COVID-19, seeking to identify ways to prevent, reduce and treat infection, and also to develop ways to effectively decontaminate exposed areas.

In Canada we also had the 'opportunity' to experiment with the bacterial agent anthrax. Occurring naturally in cattle, sheep and other animals, anthrax molecules are too big for humans to take in through our nasal hairs and pores, rendering them harmless. However, during the Second World War, British scientists found a way to weaponize anthrax, by making the spores so tiny that they could be absorbed by the human body. This process made it 300,000 times more toxic than phosgene.

The First Step

At this time anthrax was very much on all of our minds. It seemed to be the latest terrorist buzzword and leapt out of the newspaper every few months. This was mainly due to an attack just after 9/11 in which envelopes containing millions of spores were posted to addresses throughout America, including the offices of Democratic Senators Tom Daschle of South Dakota and Patrick J. Leahy of Vermont. Just fifteen spores of anthrax are enough to be deadly, so it's a miracle that this attack resulted in only five fatalities; it could have caused millions more.

However, though casualties were low it still caused plenty of terror and disruption, which was no doubt the aim. Over 30,000 people in Washington, DC, had to take prophylactic antibiotics, out of fear that they might have been infected, while extensive decontamination efforts in government buildings and post office facilities cost hundreds of millions of dollars. After a seven-year investigation, the FBI closed its case in 2008 after its chief suspect, Dr Bruce E. Ivins, a scientist at Fort Detrick, took his own life. It still amazes me that a man of science, knowing full well the affect anthrax can have, could have performed such a reckless act, especially as anthrax is so persistent. Apparently, if the British had bombed Berlin with anthrax during the Second World War, as had been considered, large parts of the city would have been uninhabitable until the 1980s.

Indeed, to my team's cost, and no little surprise, we soon found just how hot the US authorities were when it came to anthrax. One of our tasks in Canada was to work out how to weaponize naturally occurring anthrax, to allow us to understand how it worked while also helping to increase our confidence in handling such a deadly biological weapon. However, one of our team decided to 'cheat' by looking for information online. Soon after, they were arrested by the CIA and questioned, which was a little scary, if not somewhat reassuring that these things do actually get picked up by the relevant authorities.

What really scared me during this course was just how easy it seemed to be for these weapons to kill millions of unsuspecting people, whether by design or even by accident. The US Army Chemical Corps had once mounted a dummy attack on the Pentagon, one of the most secure and guarded offices in the world, prepared for all manner of attack. Despite this, operatives simply walked into the building and dropped a pint and a half of harmless bacteria into the air conditioning system, spreading it throughout the building. If the bacteria had been a deadly weapon, such as anthrax, it could have killed everyone who came into contact with it.

In 1966, the Chemical Corps Special Operations Division went one step further. They decided to mount a mock biological attack on New York City, with agents dropping bacteria through New York subway gratings. Within minutes the turbulence caused by the trains carried the bacteria throughout the tunnel system, spreading the bacteria throughout the city. It was later concluded that if anyone chose to carry out such an attack on New York, or any of the cities of the Soviet Union, Europe or South America, thousands, possibly millions would die.

Thankfully, as we were learning, it is very difficult to produce chemical and biological weapons and therefore few states or terror groups have been able to get their hands on them. However, it was rather concerning to learn about the number of accidents where they had been released.

For instance, in 1968, a fighter jet accidentally dispersed VX over Skull Valley, Utah, during a botched test. This was said to have caused the death of as a many as 6,000 sheep. If it had been released over a civilian area, its effects would have been catastrophic. Sadly, such an event occurred in 1979, when a factory in the city of Sverdlovsk, in the Soviet Union, accidentally dispersed anthrax over the local population, killing hundreds in the process.

Unsurprisingly, with this class of weapons being so dangerous, there have been multiple attempts to police and ban them since the 1925 Geneva Protocols. The latest such legislation was the Chemical Weapons Convention (CWC), which was ratified by most states, including America and Russia, in 1997.

The CWC not only banned the use and development of chemical weapons, amongst other things, but it also required all signatories to declare and destroy their stockpiles. In a far-reaching move it established an international body, the Organization for the Prohibition of Chemical Weapons (OPCW), whose 200 inspectors would be primarily responsible for enforcing the Convention, in particular ensuring the destruction of stockpiles.

However, despite all of this, it seemed the CWC and the OPCW had no place in Iraq. Owing to the fact that Iraq was not a signatory to the Convention and that coalition forces wanted to investigate for themselves, the Iraq Survey Group (ISG) was instead created to carry out the specific task of searching the country for Saddam's supposed weapons of mass destruction (WMDs). So, with my diploma under my belt, and the CBRN Regiment assigned to help the ISG, I set off for Iraq, no longer running from chemical weapons but ploughing straight for them.

4

Anthrax

It didn't take long for things in Iraq to suddenly get very real. Just weeks into the job, I was patrolling the floor of our base in Basra when I heard the nervous voice of my colleague Captain Steve Johnson.

'Sir . . .'

Turning around, I noticed a strained look on his face. Walking to his computer terminal, he glanced around before whispering under his breath, 'One of our BDSs is alarming in Umm Kasr.'

I instantly realized why he looked so worried. Biological Detection Systems (BDSs) were machines which could filter molecules of air to detect any sign of biological agents. As the molecules of these agents are larger than those found in air, the BDS could pick them up and provide us with an early report of an attack. So far, we had received no warning of any sort. In fact, I don't believe that in all the time BDSs had been in operation in the Gulf that one had ever gone off before. But that had just changed. Looking down at Johnson's screen, I saw that one of the BDSs he was monitoring had just detected anthrax. And this was no drill. This was real-world stuff. We had just been thrown straight into the deep end.

Then again, I had been in the deep end from the moment I had arrived at the British base, known as Combined Operating Base, located at what used to Basra Airport, just outside the city. On my first night, as I slept in the regiment portacabin, I was thrown out of my bed by the blast of a rocket as the camp came under attack. Thankfully, no one was killed, but apparently this was something I would have to get used to.

There was no time to ease myself in or find my feet. The world demanded to know if Saddam Hussein had WMDs, and as part of the ISG, it was the CBRN Regiment's job to help find them. After all, this was the supposed reason for the invasion, so the stakes were high. But details about these WMDs were sketchy to say the least.

It was an established fact that Saddam had previously had an arsenal of chemical weapons at his disposal. We knew that in the 1980s he had used mustard gas, sarin, tabun and VX against the Iranian Army and the Kurds, while in 1991 he had launched a chemical attack to quell a Shia revolt. Indeed, by the mid 1980s he had established the largest chemical weapons facility in the world at Al Muthana, which covered an area of 100 square kilometres.

However, following Saddam's defeat in the Gulf War, the UN Special Commission (UNSCOM) had required Iraq to declare and destroy its chemical and biological weapon stockpile, under international supervision. For Saddam, it was time to face the music. With this mandate, UNSCOM subsequently destroyed thousands of chemical munitions, but still it seemed that Saddam sought to frustrate them at every turn. UNSCOM complained of misleading declarations, concealment and acts of obstruction, amongst other things. Such was the frustration at Saddam's non-compliance that in 1998 President Bill Clinton had ordered various sites in Iraq to be bombed in Operation Desert Fox.

Despite frequent UN inspections, it was very difficult to say with any certainty whether Saddam had destroyed or given up all of his chemical weapons as had been promised. In the post-9/11 world, such deception was now deemed unacceptable to the British and American governments. Their patience had run out. Armed with intelligence that indicated that Saddam was ready to deploy his still-hidden arsenal of WMDs, the race was on to invade Iraq, topple Saddam and find the WMDs before it was too late. At the time I didn't question the politics of the invasion, or the likelihood of the WMDs being hidden in Iraq. I was just there to serve my country and do a job. If I was told to look for WMDs, that was what I was damn well going to do.

Utilizing intelligence leads and tip-offs, the CBRN Regiment searched southern Iraq high and low. We dug in the desert, stormed old factories, searched homes and even explored caves in the mountains. Despite our best efforts, we were never able to find any trace of them. But that didn't mean that they weren't still out there.

The US Army ran a programme offering up to $20,000 for the forfeiture of any chemical weapons. For some Iraqis this became a full-time profession. One farmer in particular seemed to turn up with 120mm rockets full of sarin almost every week. We would subsequently take the rockets out into the middle of the desert and blow them up, ensuring the sarin evaporated before it could do any harm.

All this was a sobering reminder that while we might not have found the so-called WMDs there were still plenty of dangerous weapons out there. Indeed, even if Saddam loyalists or other terror groups were unable to get their hands on chemical weapons, they soon learnt to improvise. Trucks carrying chlorine travelled on roads throughout Iraq every day. Chlorine was, of course, essential to filter the country's water system. In small quantities it was harmless, but the amounts carried in the container lorries could be deadly. When a tanker exploded in Anbar Province, more than a dozen people were killed and plenty more hospitalized. Whether or not this was planned or just a fortuitous mistake it's hard to say, but it certainly made the insurgents realize what could be achieved if they could destroy these tankers.

One attack in Fallujah caused as many as 350 casualties and eight deaths, as green and yellow gas clouds spread from the burning tanker into the surrounding suburbs, leaving hundreds gasping for breath. Thousands more were terrified, as the gas was not only very visual but the smell was so intense. With the vast majority having no protective masks, panic soon set in. This was the last thing we needed in a country already on a knife edge.

As well as causing terror, these attacks disrupted the supply of chlorine. There was a real concern that the country's water supply would become infected if they didn't stop. US forces struck back by raiding various warehouses in Baghdad and Anbar Province, where they found stores of lethal chemicals, propane tanks and vehicles being prepared as car bombs. However, the CBRN Regiment was also required to do its part.

In Basra, my team was instructed to put in place procedures to protect the tankers before the country was brought to a standstill. For obvious reasons, our work remains highly classified but generally this involved organizing armed guards to escort the tankers, decoys to confuse the enemy, and in some cases we even shut down roads to completely eliminate the threat. After this, no more tankers were destroyed.

However, the BDS alarming for anthrax in Umm Kasr, just thirty miles south of Basra, was the first time we faced a widespread biological attack. There had been some vicious fighting in the area in recent days, and it seemed that with Saddam's forces losing the battle they had finally unleashed our worst fears. My mind raced at the thought.

If anthrax had been used, such an attack would be disastrous. This fearsome and invisible biological pathogen could have blown for miles, over many surrounding towns and villages. The first anybody would know about being infected was in four days' time, when they would develop flu-like symptoms. By then it would already be too late. Many of our soldiers had not been vaccinated against anthrax and had also not been wearing gas masks. Thousands who had been on ops in the area could now be infected.

Research had shown that if we could treat anyone who had been infected within forty-eight hours then survival rates were excellent, at around 90%. Any later and they were as good as dead. But how on earth could we test and treat thousands of people in such a short period? As we have since seen with COVID-19, such operations can take weeks, or even months, to set up.

Another concern was what to do about the local population. We might need to test those we thought might be infected, but there was the risk that if we released this news too quickly there could be a full-blown panic. We saw such a situation in Italy during the initial COVID-19 panic. When cities in the north became infected, many fled to the south, taking the virus with them. Though this was not a virus, anthrax spores were still persistent and could travel with vehicles and people, infecting far wider areas. A full-blown humanitarian disaster would erupt, which we weren't equipped to deal with. There wasn't a second to lose.

I immediately went to see Major General Riley, who was in charge of British forces in Iraq. He didn't quite grasp the seriousness of the situation until I outlined its severity.

'General, all soldiers in the area must now be confined to base.'

'What are you talking about?' he bellowed. 'We've got them on the run. If we stop now, then they'll have the upper hand.'

'I appreciate that, sir,' I answered, 'but if these readings are correct, we could be facing thousands, if not millions of casualties. Your battalions could be wiped out.'

At this his face dropped. He was between a rock and a hard place. 'How certain are you that there has been an attack?'

'All I can go on right now, sir, is that our systems are telling us there is anthrax in the area.'

'Well, get on it, DBG! Sort it out!'

With all British forces in the area ordered to return to base, we now had to ensure we did our job as quickly as possible, before the insurgents gained the upper hand and, perhaps most importantly of all, before the anthrax spread. While my team and I had received extensive training for such an event, this was to be the first time in British Army history that it had actually been carried out in the field.

First things first. We needed to get to the area where the BDS had sounded the alarm. Looking at a map, I could see why the site might be very alluring to terrorists. Umm Kasr was the main port used by the American and British armies to ship equipment and supplies into Iraq. From there the supplies, such as food, bombs, bullets, medicines and vehicles, were taken by road to the base in Basra. The site of the BDS was just off this road, which meant that if anthrax had been used then crucial supplies would be severely disrupted, if not shut down altogether. The terrorists would effectively cut the head off the snake.

Rounding up the Command Team, we set off for the BDS in our militarized Snatch Land Rover. Alongside us was an infantry company, all wearing gas masks, while above us was a helicopter to monitor the area in case of attack. The location of the BDS was not only near a main road, which was always a threat, but it was also near an area of heavy fighting. With everyone confined to base we would be all alone. It was disconcerting to think that as of now we were the only soldiers out in the wilds of southern Iraq.

Roaring down the road, jolting in our seats thanks to the frequent potholes, I looked out of the window to see the detritus of war. The muddy terrain was littered with rubbish, while stray animals roamed free. Bombed-out, deserted buildings were the only signs of any sort of civilization. It was like something out of a *Mad Max* movie. The smell of hot garbage tingled the hairs in my nostrils. As we passed a row of power lines, I noticed that they were all bare. Thieves had stolen the copper to sell on, with no thought for the fact that the local area would now be without power. It seemed to sum up this place. Act now, think later. I just prayed that wouldn't come to define our current operation.

Every so often a rusted car would pop up in our rear-view mirror. At this our top cover, hanging out of the roof, his rifle primed, would wave for the vehicle to stay ten metres away. 'GET BACK!' he shouted. 'GET BACK NOW.' Many a soldier had already lost their life being ambushed out on the open road. It was no time to take any chances. These days, all Iraqis knew the drill, even if they didn't know the language. If anyone got too close after such a warning, they could expect to be blasted into oblivion. Every hundred yards or so the roadside was littered with the mangled remains of cars and motorbikes that had already met this fate.

As we reached our destination, my pulse rate suddenly quickened. The memory of my previous time in the Gulf

suddenly came flooding back . . . the faulty gas mask . . .
the panic . . . the gasping for breath . . . fearing I would die
. . . *Shut up!* I silently shouted at myself. *You're the commander here, so act like it!* The last thing the guys needed
was to see me fall to pieces. We had enough on our plate.

'Check your equipment, guys,' I said, trying to sound
authoritative but also acting from bitter experience. 'Make
sure your masks work and your gloves and suit are secure.'

As everyone checked themselves down, I issued a final
warning. 'If this is an anthrax attack, you can be sure we
are being watched, and right now we're the only British
soldiers in southern Iraq.' At this we all looked at each
other, with a grim sense of foreboding. 'I know we have a
job to do but keep your guns close.' Everyone nodded in
unison. Nothing more needed to be said. It was time to
move.

With the infantry and choppers surrounding us, and
with our guns by our sides, we stepped out of the Land
Rover into the searing heat of the Iraqi desert. I took in a
deep breath and instantly relaxed. The mask worked. That
was the first issue out of the way. However, it must have
been over forty degrees and our CBRN hazmat suits certainly didn't make it any cooler. Sweat was already pouring
off my forehead and fogging up my goggles, making it difficult to see. I squinted, looking this way and that for any
sign of danger: the coast appeared to be clear, for now at
least. I certainly felt comforted by the sound of the steady

hum of the helicopter blades above. If anyone came to attack us, the helicopter crew should be able to see them coming a mile off.

Waving to the guys to join me at the BDS, I couldn't help but think that in our suits, and in the barren desert, it looked as though we had landed on Mars. Everything about this place certainly felt as alien as a distant planet. Human niceties that we took as signs of civilization had been replaced here by outright evil. Just recently, American contractors had been pulled from their vehicles, torn limb from limb and their body parts put on display. At this thought my hand subconsciously wandered down to the trigger of my gun.

With my hand still on the gun, I removed the filter from the BDS so that it could be sent out to Porton Down on the next flight. Until the scientists at Porton had completed their tests we had no way of knowing what we were dealing with. It was a time-consuming process but back then this was as good as it got.

Satisfied that the area was as safe as could be, my team and I now scoured the surroundings for any sign of how the anthrax might have been dispersed. Strangely, there didn't appear to be any rocket fragments or exploded bombs in sight. If this was an attack, then it appeared the anthrax had been either sprayed from the sky or dropped from the back of a truck.

Despite this, we still had to sweep the area, taking earth and rock samples for testing. As I carefully placed a sample into a bag, I suddenly noticed, through my fogged-up lenses, a strange shape around fifty yards away. Looking closer, the shape slowly came into focus . . . *It can't be . . . but it looks like one . . .* The shape appeared to be that of a dead body. If it was, then the anthrax might have already struck. *Damn!*

'Over here!' I shouted at my team, as I quickly raced across, fearing the worst. But as I got closer, I realized that while the shape was indeed a dead body, it wasn't human. It was a camel. Still, wasn't this proof that anthrax was in the area and had killed the camel? But then something else hit me. The camel might very well have died from natural causes and then emitted naturally occurring anthrax into the air, which was not uncommon. If this was the case, the BDS might very well have picked this up. I felt a glimmer a hope at the idea. Taking a blood sample, I prayed that this might be the key to working out what was going on.

With the sample of camel blood stored in a container, I gave the order to clear out. We had all we had come for and I didn't intend to spend another minute as a sitting duck. Besides, we needed to get a move on if we were going to get the results back from Porton before the anthrax had a chance to spread. Racing to our Land Rover, we set off back to base, as a million thoughts raced through my head.

Get the samples and filter to Porton Down . . . Arrange for a shipment of antibiotics to be flown out . . . Check capacity in hospitals . . . Sort out beds and protective equipment . . .

'Brace yourselves,' one of the guys suddenly shouted. 'Enemy approaching.'

Snapping out of my to-do list, I looked behind to see a faded black truck emerge from the desert haze. Rather than slowing down at the sight of our patrol, it appeared to be picking up speed. This was unusual. The top cover in our infantry patrol waved at it to keep back but it kept on coming, hard and fast. My teeth clenched. *Slow down, you idiot. You're going to get killed.* But I wasn't too concerned for the fate of the driver at that moment, or indeed my own. All I could think about was if this idiot set off an IED he would not only kill us but also destroy the filter from the BDS. By the time the rest of the CBRN team got their act together the anthrax would be out of control. Thousands, if not millions of these idiots' countrymen would die. But there was no time to explain this. Just milliseconds remained before they took a pop at us or we took them out.

For a moment I caught sight of the driver through his dusty windshield. Just a young boy, with nothing and everything to lose. Beside him, a figure in the shadows lifted an arm, sunlight suddenly flashed off metal and then . . .

CRACK! CRACK! CRACK!

Our top cover fired his SA80 over the top of the vehicle as a warning that we were not to be messed with. I looked back; the vehicle had screeched to a halt and soon became a small speck in the distance. It was another reminder that in this hellhole you could not take your mind off the threat for one second. Perhaps we should have confronted them; they were clearly terrorists who would no doubt attack British soldiers again. But we had vital evidence that had to get back to the UK as soon as possible. The mission was to retrieve samples and at that moment this was more important than taking on a couple of the enemy.

Thirty minutes after this moment of high drama we were back at base, ensuring that before we did anything we thoroughly decontaminated ourselves and our equipment. As I said, anthrax spores are very persistent and if there had been some in the vicinity, it was very likely that we were still carrying them. After a deep clean in a chlorus solution, and with the Decontamination Team hosing our Land Rover down with disinfectant, we packed up all of our samples and had them on the next flight to Porton Down. Meanwhile, I called the Porton Operational Support Team, a group of experts on call 24/7 to aid in situations like this. Porton Down has some of the most brilliant scientific minds on the globe working in its laboratories, and, boy, was I happy that this critical 'reach back' facility was available to me. I gave them all the details and they agreed with my initial assessment that this was probably harmless anthrax from the dead camel, but I could not advise loosening the lockdown until we knew for sure.

In the meantime, I couldn't just sit back and wait for the results; I still needed to prepare for the worst. Plans were swiftly put in place to treat those infected, space was made for hospital beds, medevacs were on standby to repatriate sick soldiers and a delivery of antibiotics was waiting for the go-ahead on a runway back in the UK. We also considered potential evacuation plans for nearby towns and villages. If they were infected with anthrax, we would also need to work out how we could decontaminate them. Such an operation could take months. All the while the clock was ticking. The longer we waited for the results from Porton Down the less time we would have to react. We had only a matter of hours before we would be facing total devastation.

With Major General Riley becoming increasingly concerned at the amount of time the army was out of action, we also looked at the cost of purchasing thousands of additional gas masks, so all teams could return to operations asap. But they would take a day or two to arrive from the UK. Pressure was really ramping up now and I could sense an atmosphere of frustration setting in on the base. All eyes were on me and my team. With the clock ticking, I could wait no longer. Damn the cost, we needed the antibiotics to be flown over from the UK. We were now down to the finest of margins and any delay could cost lives.

Finally, nine hours after we had first received the reading, my phone rang. It was Porton Down. 'Shut up!' I shouted at my team, who were all frantically working away. Everyone looked at me as I answered, knowing exactly what the call was about. 'Go ahead,' I said, trying to sound calm.

'Are you sitting down, DBG?' the scientist answered, making me fear the worst. 'It was the bloody camel!'

'You're joking!' I spluttered.

'It's naturally occurring anthrax,' he laughed. 'No danger to anyone.'

Sitting back in my chair, I let out a sigh of relief. All my worst fears were over. No one was going to die. It was the ultimate result.

But not everyone was so happy . . .

'You mean to say that the whole British Army has been sat with its thumb up its arse on account of a dead camel?!' General Riley scolded.

'I'm afraid so, General,' I replied. 'But it has been an invaluable training exercise.'

I'm not sure if the general was too pleased to hear this. Thankfully, operations in the area had not been harmed too much while everyone was locked down, and the enemy was not to know that they had missed a real window of opportunity to hit us hard.

After one of the longest days of my career, I returned to my portacabin and collapsed on the bed, my tired body becoming one with the thin mattress. I reasoned that, despite the false alarm, it had been a job well done. Not only had our training, and the systems put in place, by and large worked but the top brass were also now very much aware of just how deadly and disruptive such an attack might have been.

We had also found chinks in the armour that could have cost us dearly if this *had* been real. Perhaps the biggest of these was the amount of time it took to send the samples back to Porton Down and get the results. If it had been a real attack, this could have been disastrous. For this reason, the CBRN Regiment were soon handed Polymerase Chain Reaction (PCR) machines. Initially, these machines were so large they had been confined to a lab at Porton Down, but they had now been squeezed down to the size of a printer, so that they could be used in the field. By analysing the samples' DNA ourselves, we could now find out almost instantly what we were dealing with. This was to prove a real game changer.

However, while in this instance my training had somewhat helped me rise to the occasion, I was soon to face a real threat: one of the most dangerous military operations the British Army has ever known, for which there was no textbook.

5

The Bomb

By 2008 Afghanistan supplied more than 90% of the world's opium, providing billions of dollars to Afghan officials, insurgents, drug traffickers, warlords and the Taliban. It also provided millions of jobs and was such a booming trade that it was estimated that heroin was responsible for 52% of the country's GDP. For the people of Afghanistan, this industry was vital. For the Americans, and the rest of the world, it was a scourge that had to be stamped out.

Amazingly, this boom in heroin production had only occurred after the 2001 US invasion. The subsequent collapse of the economy, and the scarcity of other sources of revenue, forced many of the country's farmers to diversify their crop and grow opium, readily encouraged by Taliban insurgents, who required significant funding to fight the US occupation. With farmers able to make one hundred times more money growing opium than wheat, it was a no-brainer for them.

The Bomb

Afghanistan's opium production subsequently surged from around 180 tonnes in 2001 to more than 3,000 tonnes a year after the invasion. By 2007 it was producing over 8,000 tonnes. The country had truly become a narco-state. Every spring, the opium harvest would fill the Taliban's coffers, funding wages for a new crop of guerrilla fighters, who were each paid an average of $300 (US) a month – far above the wages they would have made as agricultural labourers, ensuring their loyalty to the cause.

Helmand Province was a particularly valuable region to the Taliban. Thanks to the Helmand River, which irrigated mile upon mile of poppy fields, it was a pivotal cog in the Afghan drug machine, producing 66% of the country's poppy output in 2008 alone. With the Taliban regrouping and looking to retake the country, coalition forces had to act fast. A series of military operations were conducted by the International Security Assistance Force (ISAF), which mostly consisted of British soldiers, against Taliban insurgents and opium producers, aiming to eradicate the poppy crop and bring the Taliban to its knees. Unsurprisingly, the Taliban did not take this lying down and vicious fighting broke out all over the region.

So what did all this have to do with me, you might ask? Well, after two years commanding the CBRN Regiment, and then NATO's Rapid Reaction CBRN Battalion, my time in the role was at an end. I had loved commanding the regiment, not only the day-to-day stuff in Iraq, searching for and destroying chemical weapons, but also working with other CBRN teams around the world, with many of our operations still classified. It was also a thrill to speak to some of the world's greatest scientists at Porton Down every day, which really advanced my understanding and knowledge far more than any degree could have. Commanding NATO's Rapid Reaction CBRN Battalion was also a real honour. While we didn't see any action, it was still an important role, commanding a team made up of different nationalities and training them in Portugal, Poland and the UK. From having no interest in the subject at all, I had come to be considered one of NATO's top CBRN men, which made me very proud. I had been surprised at just how much I had enjoyed the role and was sorry to leave, but it was now time for me to move on, as is so often the case in the military. You get your feet under the table in one role, and then it's on to the next.

However, though I was pleased to be made a colonel, I was very disappointed to find that I was not immediately selected for the Higher Command and Staff Course, which would have allowed me to command at brigade level and above. Passing this course would have been the silver bullet to the big leagues, but instead I was told, 'Bide your time, DBG. You still need a bit more experience.'

This was extremely frustrating but in 2008 I received an intriguing call from Paddy Allison, the head of Intelligence, Surveillance and Target Acquisition and Reconnaissance

The Bomb

(ISTAR). He asked if I would be his deputy, which I must admit seemed a sideways move after my stint commanding the CBRN Regiment, but Paddy certainly did a good job of selling it to me.

'This is a little different to what you've been doing in Iraq,' he warned, 'but I think you'll have fun.' It turned out to be *very* different to what I had been doing previously. In fact, there was no link to CBRN at all, which I found to be a little disappointing, after all I had learnt, but it still seemed to be very exciting.

My role primarily entailed overseeing the drawing of information from a variety of overt and covert sources, such as drones and reconnaissance forces. This information would help provide the intelligence needed to support military operations and contingency planning, as well as to inform defence policy and procurement decisions.

Much of the role would be split between Army HQ in the UK and Afghanistan, which suited me perfectly, as I would be able to spend much more time with Julia and the kids. Having already missed chunks of Jemima and Felix's childhood, thanks to my excursions in Iraq and beyond, I felt this change was important. Some time at home would also allow me to remember what normal life was actually like. Everything in Iraq had been a thousand miles an hour, so this new role gave me a chance to catch my breath and be part of the family, doing regular things like eating out, going to the cinema and crashing out on the sofa together.

Then, when I was back in Afghanistan, it would be all systems go again.

In order to get my teeth into the role, I was first sent to Afghanistan in 2008 to get some experience of ISTAR's 'dynamic or precision' targeting programme. If you've seen the terrific Helen Mirren film *Eye in the Sky*, you might know what this entails. An aircraft, usually a Nimrod in those days, flying at 20,000 feet, carried a powerful camera that can track terrorists in the most unbelievable detail. It was mind-blowing how advanced the technology was, even back then. If someone was eating a chocolate bar, we could probably tell what brand it was. This level of accuracy made a huge difference to our counter-insurgency work.

The footage from the Nimrod would be instantaneously relayed to the ops room, where my team and I would monitor the feed from our base at Lashkargah, the capital of Helmand Province, where most of the opium war was now taking place. Our primary aim was to disrupt the drug trade by cutting off the Taliban's funding, and limiting the amount of drugs that reached British shores in the process. As such, most of our targets were usually linked to the drug industry in some way, whether they were producers, dealers, warlords or important figures in the Taliban. We could follow them from the bright red poppy fields around the Helmand River all the way back to their homes, then pick an opportune time to order a precision strike with a smart bomb. These bombs could track a target even when they were on the move or changed course. But more often than not, our targets didn't know what was coming. The system was unbelievably accurate and merciless.

From the comfort of your chair it almost felt like a computer game, watching a target come up on screen and then, within a blink of an eye, there was just a black smudge where there had once been life. Being so far removed from the action, and not being able to see the whites of the enemy's eyes before they were killed, was a strange sensation. In fact, watching it, I almost felt nothing at all. All the operators had to do was click a button and they were dead, all with no threat whatsoever to me or my team. Whether I would have felt differently if we had killed them face to face I can't be sure, although I must admit I didn't lose much sleep over them. These guys were total scumbags who had brought misery to their country as well as the rest of the world, heroin use having exploded. I appreciate that this may seem rather cold, but it's the truth. But I almost couldn't comprehend that what we were seeing on the screen was real, that real people were dying. Something in my brain just couldn't connect the two. That's the only way I can describe it.

Lately, things in Helmand had been getting a little hairy. Just a few months before, in May 2008, the Taliban had launched attacks on towns just 10 kilometres from our camp. By September the towns were pretty much theirs, with the Taliban said to have received plenty of local support due to promising to eradicate the coalition's poppy programmes. Next in their sights was Lashkargah itself.

While things outside the camp might have been getting tense, it was pretty quiet for us on the base, which I sought to take full advantage of. A typical day saw me up at dawn to hit the gym, where I'd sweat buckets as the temperature steadily hit 40 degrees. I would then work in HQ until 11 p.m. every night, crunching the latest intel and tracking targets, before treating myself to a cigar under the stars. Despite my initial disappointment when I took on the role, I was having a good time, so much so that I christened the camp the 'Lashkargah Health Spa'. After working hard and training hard, I was soon pretty ripped and thoroughly enjoying myself. I didn't even feel as if I was in war zone. But things were swiftly turned on their head.

In June 2008, as we were monitoring the feed, I heard the distant sound of an explosion. Word soon reached us that our worst fears had been realized: the Taliban was launching a direct attack on Lashkargah itself. Climbing to the roof of a portacabin, I looked out on to the city, which was less than a mile away. It looked like Fireworks Night out there. Hundreds of Taliban militia were bombarding the city from three sides, with tracers and mortars lighting up the sky, screeching and booming. Down below, soldiers and jeeps all scurried into action, ready to defend the city as well as the camp itself. Orders were being barked, weapons were being prepared. It was clear things were going to get pretty nasty out there.

I was just about to return to my post, as no doubt ISTAR would be needed to pick out targets, when a voice came from the shadows, 'Colonel de Bretton-Gordon?' I turned to find what I can only describe as a very nondescript man: average build with an unremarkable face. Wearing a cream cotton suit, he made me think of the Man from Del Monte. From my previous experience of dealing with such people, I instantly took him to be a spook.

'You have just finished commanding the Joint CBRN Regiment, is that correct?' he asked.

'Yes,' I replied, wondering where this was going, as another rocket hit its target in the distance, lighting the city with an orange glow.

'I'm with the British Embassy Drugs Team. We have a problem and we need your help.'

This sounded pretty ominous. The BEDT was a sort of euphemism for MI6, and their main role in Afghanistan was to take down the drugs trade. But what on earth had this to do with me? I was soon to find out.

'There was a raid on an opium factory,' he revealed – this was no doubt one of the reasons the Taliban was now pushing so hard in Lashkargah. 'The police confiscated the containers from the laboratories and stored them in their cellar, but we are very concerned.'

'How do you mean?'

'The bottles are leaking on to each other. We are not really sure what we are dealing with but it doesn't smell or look good. We need an expert to take a look, and as it stands, you are the top CBRN man in the area.'

'Crikey . . . *Am I?*'

From the tone of his voice it was clear that there was no time to hang around. War zone or no war zone, this required urgent attention. Yet before we could go, I needed some protective equipment. If things were as dangerous as he suspected, I couldn't just walk in bareback. But other than a respirator, I didn't have anything with me. So I made a quick trip to the Quartermaster, who, despite the chaos, was able to conjure up a pair of wellingtons and some rubber gloves, while I also put on extra desert combats as a sacrificial layer. It was far from perfect but for now it would have to do.

We jumped into the spook's car, drove out through the camp gates and made our way to the police station, which was less than a mile away. However, leaving the safety of the camp was like stepping into another world. I had rarely set foot in the town, even when things were quiet, but now, out in the open, I could really get a sense of just what our soldiers were up against. As the glow of the occasional mortar lit our way, I could see that the city was a sprawl of two-level buildings, set out in grids for as far as the eye could see. Everywhere I looked there was pandemonium. People were shouting and screaming, running to safety or to take up attack positions; whether they were British soldiers or the Taliban I had no idea. But I knew I would feel a lot safer once we were under cover.

As we drove, we passed two mangled cars in the middle of the road, their drivers in an escalating argument to apportion blame, ignoring the ever-growing cacophony of war. Horns of other cars incessantly beeped at them, as the streetlights flickered on and off, freezing their agitated faces before enveloping them in darkness. I felt as if I was in Saigon at the end of *The Deer Hunter*, just before the city fell. But rather than rescuing Christopher Walken from a game of Russian roulette, I would soon be playing my own deadly game.

In a little under five minutes we pulled up at the police station, which I saw was under heavy armed guard. In the cells were several valuable Taliban assets, not to mention items confiscated from the raid, and there was a real fear that if the Taliban broke through, they would storm the station, killing anyone who stood in their way. As I got out of the car, the smell of black smoke hit my nostrils, the result of a fire a few blocks away. The spook nodded to the guards, who instantly stepped out of his way, allowing us to pass.

Inside the station an Afghan police officer quickly approached us, fraught and frantic.

'Is this the man?' he said, looking at me. The spook nodded, then turned to me.

'The door is over there,' he said, gesturing in the direction of the cellar. Walking across, I opened the door only to instantly recoil.

'Bloody hell' I coughed, as the overpowering smell of chemicals sent me spluttering backwards. The spook stared at me with a knowing look: 'Told you so.' The situation was clearly as dangerous as he had made out.

As I put on my respirator, the Afghan police officer said he wanted to go down with me, but as he did not have a gas mask I told him to stay put.

'I do not need a mask. I am a brave man,' he shouted.

'That may be the case but if you go down there without one, you won't be brave for very long.'

This stopped him in his tracks. Judging by the strength of the smell, it was a miracle that the men in the police station were not already seriously ill.

As I made my way slowly down the steps the room suddenly opened up before me. There, lit by a lone flicking bulb, was a tremendous sight. Though there were six huge bags of brown heroin – which would have had a street value of about $10million – I barely paid any notice of them. What really grabbed my attention was the countless blue 20l containers stacked up against the walls.

Kneeling in front of one, I noticed that all the seals were broken, hence the smell. Careful not to spill anything, I wiped away the dirt on one of the labels. The words 'Sulphuric Acid' appeared. Moving quickly, I did the same to the next container, and the next. The labels revealed a mixture of 'Hydrochloric Acid', 'Hydrogen Peroxide', 'Ether' and 'Sodium Chloride'. Some containers had no labels at all, but the contents were clearly highly volatile.

My heart stopped. This wasn't good. In fact, it was a major disaster waiting to happen. I quickly worked out that we had about 54 tonnes of leaking acid and alkaline in the cellar. The acid alone would have been cause for concern but together with the leaking alkaline there were the perfect materials for a huge fertilizer bomb. To put this into perspective, the bomb used in the 2017 Manchester Arena attack contained a kilogram of explosive, whereas the chemicals in the cellar were enough for 54,000 kilograms. All it needed was a spark.

As I tried to gather myself and work out a plan of action, the room vibrated with the impact of a distant explosion. A chill ran through me. We needed to get these chemicals out of the cellar as a matter of urgency. There was no time to waste.

Back upstairs, I saw the spook and his Afghan colleague were anxiously waiting for me. I think my grave face told its own story. 'I . . . I need to speak to a few people,' I said, trying to ensure my voice did not betray my shaking nerves.

Calling the Porton Down emergency line, I breathlessly told them just what we were facing. While Porton Down deal with major situations on a regular basis, and the staff are always calm and collected, I think this caused them to take a deep breath. It was a situation report to flip the stomach. Rapidly producing a HPAC spread, to show the likelihood of death and injury if the place did go up, they revealed the downwind hazard from the police station was straight through the city, as well as the British camp. Hundreds of thousands of people could die. Goosebumps prickled my skin. It would obliterate us all.

Without a second to lose I called Brigade Commander John Lorimer, an old friend, and told him of the threat we were facing. Unsurprisingly, he was preoccupied with keeping the Taliban at bay but he was certainly clear with his orders: 'Get that stuff out of harm's way pronto, DBG!' But how the hell were we going to get this stuff out of the station and then dispose of it?

Keeping in touch with the experts at Porton Down, I suggested mixing the acids and the alkalis together, which would produce a pH7 solution and make the chemicals neutral. This seemed to be a good option. But combining them together like this could make the mix extremely unstable. One wrong move and it would blow up in our faces. To make this work, we needed a large amount of water to cool it down, and this was certainly something the police station was not equipped for.

However, in these conditions, there was no way we could risk taking the chemicals very far. I had already seen myself just how chaotic it was outside. Even a heavily armed ops team, or air support, to protect the chemical load would be of little use. British army vehicles, surrounded by massive firepower from all sides, would effectively raise a red flag. It would be quite clear to the enemy that we were transporting something of monumental importance and they would try to attack. Even if the ops teams were able to destroy any enemies who crossed our path, if just one of their rockets, bombs or bullets hit our truck then everything would be wiped out. It was therefore vital that we kept as low profile as possible.

It seemed there was only one solution. The British base was in the northern suburbs of the city, just a short journey away. We had to get the chemicals inside the base and do the mix there. Taking a highly explosive bomb into the heart of the British forces during a major conflict was hardly the best idea, but what other choice did we have? We couldn't leave the chemicals where they were, nor could we risk trying to transport them out of the city. The army base was our only option, as dangerous as it may be.

However, to mix the chemicals we needed a huge mixing tank, with three openings in the top to pour in the acids, alkalis and water separately. Calling the Quartermaster, I told him what I required, shouting over the ever-growing noise of the fighting outside. He said he would get on it right away.

While he did this, we had to move the chemicals. The longer they were left in the police station the more we were all in danger. But what could we move them in? The spook's car certainly wouldn't suffice.

'Do you have any trucks?' I asked the Afghan policeman.

'Yes,' he nodded. 'We have one.'

'Is it big enough to fit all of the chemicals?'

'Yes, we brought them all here in it in the first place,' he answered.

This was a start, although I certainly would have preferred not to have to travel in a marked police truck when we needed to keep a low profile. But I would worry about that later; for now we needed to get moving. I looked at the spook and the policeman. 'OK, this is the plan . . .'

As I was the only one with a respirator and any protective equipment, I moved the containers from the basement to the top of the stairs. From there, the spook and the policeman loaded them on to the truck. There was a huge amount to get through, and each container was very heavy, and they felt even more so carrying them up the stairs in a building without air conditioning. But for now this was my focus, container after container, step after step. I blocked out all of the noise outside and all my worries. Nothing could get in my way. I remembered my Sandhurst instructor – a man who had fought in the Falklands with the Welsh Guards – and was grateful for the motto he had drilled into us from dawn to dusk: 'Fitness will see you through, sirs.' Finally, all those hours in the gym and pounding the hills paid off. I had to act like a machine. No thoughts. No emotions. Just get those bloody containers out of the building as quickly as we could.

But in my haste I tripped, dropping an unmarked container, allowing a drop of its contents to leak on to my wellington boot. Looking down, I saw that it had burnt a hole right through the rubber. If one drop could do that, then what the whole container could do to the human body didn't bear thinking about.

After two hours of this relentless, back-breaking work, I had almost managed to forget the escalating conflict outside. Until a cry came from the top of the stairs: 'The Taliban . . . They can't keep them away much longer.'

I looked up to the top of the stairs. The Afghan policeman was urging me to hurry.

'How much time do we have?' I shouted.

'Twenty minutes, maybe less,' he cried.

I looked around the cellar. There was no way I could clear it by myself in that time, and there was certainly no way we could leave the rest of the chemicals behind.

'All right,' I shouted. 'Cover your faces and get down here. I'm going to need your help.'

At this the policeman and the spook raced down. It was a gamble, but with most of the containers already removed, I hoped that they wouldn't be overcome by the remaining fumes as we desperately moved the containers to the truck.

Stepping out of the station at last, the humid air buffeting my skin, I heard a round of gunshots fill the air.

Pow! Pow! Pow!

I had no idea who was firing but it was a reminder of just how quickly we now had to move, especially as most of the chemicals were now in the truck, and it was out in the open, at the police station no less. Just one stray gunshot and we would all be goners.

'Hurry!' I shouted, as the policeman and the spook carried up the last of the containers and loaded them inside, both panting and wheezing, soaked through with sweat. As the spook and I jumped into the truck, I thanked the policeman for his help. Without him we would have been really up against it. '*Inshallah*,' he replied, shaking my hand. But now we both had very separate missions. He had to protect the station, while we faced the most hazardous part of our operation, taking this huge fertilizer bomb back to base in the middle of a war zone.

Apart from the mayhem of being in the middle of a battle, our initial journey to the station had been relatively uneventful and had taken less than five minutes. Now it was a different matter entirely. Any spark or bullet was liable to kill us, taking most of those in the city, not to mention our colleagues in the British base, along with us. We just couldn't risk going anywhere near any heavy fighting. And so this time we had to take an indirect route.

While this should avoid the fighting, it would also leave us out in the open even longer.

Weaving in and out of dark alleyways, the muffled sounds of more explosions and gunshots seemingly all around us, we suddenly jolted to a stop at a junction. Passing us on the main road was a convoy of trucks, all carrying Afghans on the back brandishing various weapons. As two Westerners driving an Afghan police truck, we knew we were bound to attract attention; we had to keep a low profile at the best of times, let alone now.

'What do you think?' the spook whispered. 'Taliban?'

It was hard to say. I had no idea who was friend or foe. The men on the truck, scouring the area, ready to strike at any moment, could very well have been our allies, patrolling the streets for Taliban, but we could not take that risk. By this stage many Afghans were openly hostile towards British soldiers. Thousands had already been killed in the most horrendous manner. This was a thought that certainly quickened the pulse. The Taliban would love nothing more than a British soldier and a spook to torture and parade as trophies. We had to play it as safe as we could.

Nervous tension built as we waited in silence, holding our breath, watching the convoy pass. Finally, there was an opening. Shooting out of the alleyway, and across the junction, we entered another labyrinth, only to find more vehicles heading towards us. 'That way!' I shouted, as the spook spun the truck 180 degrees and moved into another warren of alleyways. Looking over my shoulder, I saw that one of the vehicles was behind us.

'Are they following us?' I asked. The spook glanced into his rear-view mirror, as my fingers twitched towards the gun in my belt.

'One way to find out,' he said as he jerked the truck hard left, leaving the vehicle behind.

For a few moments we drove in silence, both glancing back to see if the vehicle would follow.

'Is it gone?' the spook asked.

'Looks like it,' I said, taking a deep breath. It seemed paranoia had got the better of us.

'How much further?' I asked, totally disorientated by the darkness and the roundabout route, occasionally lit up by the spectral visuals of war.

'Just a few minutes.'

Travelling onwards, apparently out of harm's way, a noisy roar of heavy gunfire suddenly surrounded us, sending the truck careering into the side of a wall.

As the truck ground to a halt, black smoke pouring out of the engine, gunfire seemed to be coming from all angles. Such was the deafening noise it seemed a miracle we had not yet been hit.

'Get us away from here!' I shouted, adrenalin running through me. But as the spook turned the keys, the engine only coughed and spluttered.

The Bomb

'It won't start,' he said, turning the keys again and again, more black smoke spiralling into the air while around us silhouettes of men running to and fro plastered the sand-coloured walls. Panic gripped my chest. If we couldn't get going soon, our load was going to be hit or – best-case scenario – we would be dragged from the truck and killed.

'Try it again,' I cried, not knowing what else to say or do, other than open the window, ready to shoot anyone who approached. Again, the engine coughed and spluttered. Again, it failed to start. *We've had it,* I thought, watching stray gunshots spit chunks of granite out of a nearby wall, when suddenly . . .

Vroom . . . VROOM!

The engine revved and kicked into action. 'Go! Go! Go!' I cried, as the truck violently jolted forward. Screeching and whining, the truck couldn't go any faster than twenty miles an hour but it at least got us away from the heavy fighting. I just prayed it had enough left in it to get us back to base.

'How much further?' I asked again, not sure we were going to make it.

'Just a few minutes,' came the response, as more black smoke from our engine filled the air, making me worry that the truck could catch fire, setting the chemicals alight in the process. Would this ordeal ever end?

Minutes later we trundled up to the gates of the base. Flashing our credentials to the guards on patrol, we were waved inside to relative safety. To say it had been a white-knuckle ride so far was an understatement. Yet there was still a lot of hard work ahead of us.

The time was now just past 1.30 a.m. If all went well, I hoped to have disposed of the chemicals and neutralized the threat by 7 a.m. at the latest. Stashing the chemicals in the furthest corner of the base, and downwind, we went to the Quartermaster, praying he had somehow managed to conjure up a mixing tank.

To my relief, the Quartermaster presented us with a good-looking tank, which we proceeded to position on a flatbed trailer. At around 3 a.m., with the tank in position at the mixing site at the back of the camp, we finally got to work. From here, the sound of the bombs and gunshots going off in the city were muffled. We could at least work without too much risk of being hit. But nothing came easy to us. In the interim, I had received an urgent message from Porton Down: 'DO NOT MIX IN TEMPERATURES OVER 30 DEGREES. MIXTURE COULD EXPLODE.'

Even at 3 a.m. the temperature was hovering around 25 degrees. By 6 a.m. it would be close to the danger zone. So we had less than three hours to synthesize the lot, all the while hoping it wouldn't blow up in our faces. If we delayed, the risk of explosion would be too high. Time for a herculean effort.

Putting on our makeshift protective suits and gas masks, I realised that Porton Down recommended only wearing a mask in these temperatures for a few minutes; three hours was therefore going to be very tough. Sweating buckets, we steadily moved our way through the containers, loading the acid and alkaline into our mixing tank, while an army water truck filled the main tank to keep it cool.

Though we were facing a race against time, we couldn't rush the process – I'd already seen what happened when I had spilt a drop on my boots. We needed to be quick but careful, yet at this point I had been up for twenty-four hours. Fatigue was well and truly setting in. But with the sun starting to rise over the horizon, I saw that the temperature gauge on one of our thermometers had hit 28 degrees.

'Faster,' I shouted. 'We don't have much time.'

We were now reaching the critical point. With each container we emptied into the tank we ran the risk of it exploding, but the last thing we wanted was for this to go on any longer. We had to neutralize the lot now. Even with most of the chemicals neutralized, there was still enough left to take out a chunk of the base. And there was certainly enough left to kill the two of us.

Powering through, we ignored the tiredness, the heat, the sound of mortars exploding in the distance, and our aching muscles. Minute after minute we emptied more and more containers into the bowl, being careful to add equal amounts. The spook let out a cry as a drop spilt on his arm, leaving him with a nasty burn. He swore loudly, to no one in particular, venting his frustration, before getting back down to work. I took a quick look at my watch: 5.45. The temperature was now 29 degrees.

'We should stop,' the spook warned. 'We shouldn't risk it.'

I looked at what we had left. With one last push, I thought we could do it and end this nightmare once and for all.

'Come on,' I shouted. 'Just a few more.'

As the temperature hovered between 29 and 30 degrees, I didn't take my eyes off the thermometer. Any further increase in temperature and I knew we would have to call it a day, but it held firm on 29 degrees as we finally mixed the last of the 20,000 gallons. We now had a non-volatile pH7 solution that could be safely disposed of.

Our work wasn't over yet, though: we still needed to get rid of fifty large glass bottles of ether that were at risk of combusting when the temperature reached 32 degrees. With the sun well and truly up, and the temperature climbing past 30 already, I had an unconventional but effective idea. Placing the bottles on the Hesco bastion that surrounded the camp, we removed their tops and retreated to a safe location, waiting for the searing sun to work its magic . . .

BANG! BANG! BANG!

One after the other they exploded, spraying fragments of glass as far as fifty metres, causing us to put our arms over our heads to protect ourselves.

The Bomb

When the last one finally exploded, I sank on to my haunches, totally exhausted. My clothes were soaked with sweat while the skin on my lips was parched. I hadn't had a drop of water since I'd left the camp last night. As the sun rose, the spook and I sat on the dusty floor, puffing and panting. A major disaster had been averted and we had escaped by the skin of our teeth, but by God it had been close.

While we had done our part to keep the city and the camp safe, our colleagues had been hard at work doing likewise, repelling the Taliban insurgents with a series of deadly air strikes, killing their leader Mullah Qudratullah in the process. The police station was also safe. All in all, I don't think we could have asked for a better outcome. The camp and the town were out of harm's way and 10 million dollars' worth of heroin was off the streets. In my remaining time in Lashkargah, the Taliban never again attempted to take the city. But if I thought my chemical adventures in Afghanistan were now at an end, I was wrong. Another issue soon reared its head, one that was to flip my career, and life, upside down.

6

Convictions

As a British patrol passed through a series of Afghan villages, all seemed well. Conditions were clear, there was no Taliban in sight and the villagers did not appear to be particularly threatening. This was as good as things could get in a country where patrols were regularly ambushed and where in 2009 alone over 100 British soldiers had already lost their lives in this manner. Yet as the patrol turned a corner, they suddenly realized all of the villagers had gone inside. Something was clearly up.

From the roof of a Land Rover, the top cover spotted someone from the corner of his eye. 'Stop!' he shouted, ready to squeeze the trigger of his gun. But it was already too late. At that moment an IED was set off, shredding the metal of the Land Rover and throwing it across the road, as a child might throw away a toy. Two of the soldiers inside died instantly – one was just twenty-one years of age. Another was severely wounded. Just three young men, serving their country, and in a blink of an eye it was all over.

At this time I was still Deputy Director of ISTAR, with no invitation to sit the Higher Command and Staff Course in sight. I was now forty-six and feeling that my dreams were slowly but surely inching away from my grasp. Once more I was told to bide my time, but time was surely running out. Indeed, I had always dreaded the thought of being stuck behind a desk and this role certainly provided plenty of that, albeit in between pockets of excitement.

Though I was now primarily based at Army HQ in the UK, I was frequently sent on trips to Camp Bastion in Afghanistan, a massive base situated in the middle of the desert. There I continued to monitor a variety of overt and covert sources to help provide intelligence to the powers that be. As I said in the previous chapter, the drones were especially effective in this regard. The footage they sent back was incredibly clear and allowed us to follow our targets, keeping track of them at all times. Reconnaissance forces allowed us to fill in the blanks. They typically collected intelligence from captured insurgents, either by interview or by scouring through their mobile phones, computers and other personal items. This was often crucial. We usually found a mother lode of information on phones or computer records, detailing associates, potential targets and operation plans, as well as hide-out locations. With all this, we were able to round up more of the enemy and bring them to justice, sometimes stopping attacks before they had even happened. This was yet another reminder that in modern warfare the tank was becoming increasingly obsolete. In places like Afghanistan, bombs and bullets will only get you so far.

British patrols being hit by roadside bombs was sadly an occupational hazard in Afghanistan. If anything, things seemed to be getting worse. In the two years I had been in and out of the country I had almost grown immune to the relentless brutality. On one occasion a child had crossed a patrol's path while pushing a wheelbarrow. When the patrol stopped to allow the child to pass, its parents, who were hiding out of sight, set off a bomb hidden in the wheelbarrow, killing all those on patrol but also their own child. This sort of atrocity was becoming run of the mill as the country continued to sink into the depths of depravity.

There were many aspects to my role, but I found nothing more satisfying than helping find those who were responsible for such crimes and ensuring that they spent the rest of their days behind bars. This occasion was no different. The young men who had been killed or injured were on their first tours. I thought of my time in the Gulf War and how I might have met a similar fate, never having the opportunity to marry Julia, have two beautiful children and travel the world with the army. I also thought of the boys' poor families. They would now have to say goodbye to their sons before their lives had really had a chance to blossom. It really stuck in my throat. They had signed up to defend their country, only to be killed by gutless cowards.

The intelligence team I worked with in Bastion were brilliant and were all exceptionally well-drilled. I told them that the very least we could do to honour these soldiers was to find their killers and ensure they got the punishment they deserved. A lifetime in jail certainly did not equate to the vicious crime that had been committed but in the circumstances that was as much as we could do.

For the next few days, the team interrogated prisoners, interviewed villagers, searched phone records to try to pinpoint who might have been in the area at the time, and collected fragments from the bomb to study. All the evidence indicated the involvement of one of the most wanted men in Afghanistan, a high-value target known as Mohammed Abdullah (for security reasons I am unable to reveal the man's real name, therefore this is a pseudonym).

It was thought that Abdullah was responsible for organizing the making of many of the bombs that had killed British soldiers in the region. The team had brought him into custody before but had not managed to build a strong enough case with which to charge him. As much as it had stuck in everyone's throats, they had had no choice but to release him, upon which he had disappeared into the mountains, where he had continued to make bombs to murder and maim. But now the team's hard work had revealed where he might be hiding, and they were determined that we were not going to allow him to slip through our hands again.

In the middle of the night, British special forces descended on his small village bolthole. Banging down the door, they dragged Abdullah from his bed as he reached for his gun. Moments later he was being hauled on to a helicopter in handcuffs and taken to Camp Bastion. By the morning he was sitting in the interrogation room, refusing to answer any questions, even to confirm his own name.

'Look at him,' a colleague snarled behind one-sided glass. 'No remorse whatsoever!'

'What have we got on him so far?' I asked.

'His phone records show he was in the area. Witnesses have verified this, and the bomb is consistent with others he's made.'

This was all well and good but it was still just circumstantial. To really nail him, we needed something far harder-hitting, especially if we were going to prove to an Afghan court that he was guilty.

'Do we have a sample of his DNA yet?' I asked, to which my colleague shook his head. 'Take a swab,' I requested, knowing this might be all we could rely on.

As Abdullah had previously been in custody, he knew the drill. Military law decreed that we had four days to question and charge him. If we were unable to do this within that time, he would again walk free. No matter what threats or incentives we threw his way, there was fat chance he would say a word to us. All he had to do was sit tight and wait for the time to run out. I hoped DNA evidence might change all that.

We all leave traces of our individual DNA on whatever we touch. In some cases we don't even need to touch an item for our DNA to be found on it. DNA can travel in saliva droplets when we talk or from a cough or a sneeze. We also shed 50 million skin cells a day, which can fall on an object we haven't physically touched. Therefore, if you can link someone's unique DNA to a particular item, then at some point they would at the very least have to have been near that item. The detection of DNA traces had revolutionized the criminal justice system over the course of the last decade and it was certainly something we looked to take advantage of.

If Abdullah had touched the bomb, or had been near it, then even though it had exploded, the fragments we had recovered could still contain traces of his DNA. It was therefore vitally important to get the fragments tested alongside a sample. But I was already well aware of a problem. We would need to send the samples back to Porton Down, and the current guidance stated that the test results would take fourteen days. We clearly could not wait that long.

Calling Porton Down, I described the situation, in the hope that something could be done.

'I know we usually have to wait fourteen days for DNA results,' I said, 'but if we don't get a match within the next twenty-four hours, then we'll have to release one of the most wanted men in Afghanistan.'

'I appreciate that,' came the reply. 'But there's nothing I can do. We already have a backlog of important requests.'

The system was crazy. By the time we had a match this murderous thug would have been released, free to disappear and continue to wreak havoc. I knew there were rules we had to abide by – after all, that's what separated us from the likes of Abdullah – but I thought much more could be done in a case like this. How were British soldiers meant to feel? I know that if I were out there risking my life every day, I would want to know that I had the full support of my country, who would move heaven and earth to get me justice.

As the minutes ticked by, I sat at my desk running the scenario over and over in my head. We somehow needed to jumpstart the DNA analysis and boil down what usually took fourteen days into just a few hours. Far easier said than done, of course. The only experience I had with DNA was with the CBRN Regiment, where we had used Polymerase Chain Reaction (PCR) machines to find if a sample contained a biological agent by analysing the unique DNA structures of specific agents, like anthrax. Suddenly it hit me. If PCR machines could identify the DNA of a biological agent, maybe the same process would work on a human sample? And we already had the machines here, in Afghanistan. Yet this all seemed too easy. Surely some-one must have thought of this already?

Grabbing the phone, I called my boss, Brigadier Paddy Allison, and hurriedly explained my idea, fully expecting to be shot down.

There was a long pause. Finally, the response came: 'That just might work.' At the very least it had to be worth a shot. It was all we had.

By now there were just sixteen hours remaining until Abdullah would have to be released. We had to move fast. As the PCR machine arrived at base, the intel guys swiftly took the sample of Abdullah's DNA and ran it through the machine, along with samples from the frag-ments of the bomb. The entire case against Abdullah hinged on there being a match. Without it, we would have to let him go.

Suddenly, one of the intel team turned to me, grinning. 'Abdullah is our man!' Intense relief swept over me. With this match we could now officially charge him. But for some reason the intel team leader didn't seem to share my elation when I told him.

'I've been speaking to legal about this,' he said, with a hint of trepidation in his voice. 'They don't think DNA evidence will stand up in an Afghan court.'

'What are you talking about?' I argued. 'DNA is the best evidence you can get.'

'We know that, and our courts know that, but Afghan courts are not used to working with DNA analysis. It's not currently recognized as a legitimate form of evidence.'

To their credit, we had found the judges in Afghanistan to be very educated and fair. But due to Taliban restrictions they were unsurprisingly behind the rest of the world in some matters. They were catching up all the time but as yet had not got as far as DNA. Another issue we faced was that we had sourced the DNA match from a machine that had not been strictly designed for this purpose. It was surely something that any decent lawyer would challenge in court.

My heart sank. There were now only three hours until Abdullah was to be released. It appeared we were all out of luck, and ideas. The team and I were totally demoralized. We knew this guy was guilty beyond all reasonable doubt but all that would keep him in custody now was a confession, which we were very unlikely to get. But as dismay set in, one of the team suddenly stood up.

'Abdullah knows we were checking his DNA for a match . . .'

'So what? He probably doesn't even know what DNA is!' another of my team replied.

'Yes, but he knows he's guilty and he doesn't know how the DNA-match procedure works.'

'What are you saying?' I asked, suddenly intrigued.

'Let's show him that the match is positive. Then see what he does.'

We all looked at each other, suddenly hopeful. In the absence of all other options it was a bloody good shout. But I was concerned that Abdullah might not understand the PCR machine results. We needed something simple, something that he could see with his own eyes and grasp instantly. At this, one of the team had an idea.

Taking a laptop into the interrogation room, the translator explained to Abdullah that we needed him to place his fingerprint on to the screen, to see if there was a match to the sample we had collected from the bomb. If there wasn't a match, he could go free, but if he didn't touch the screen, we could charge him anyway.

It was Catch-22. All of a sudden, his cocky demeanour disappeared. He knew full well he was in real trouble now, but he had no choice but to comply. Slowly he raised his finger and as he touched the screen it was remotely changed (at this time, of course, touchscreens were very much in their infancy). Suddenly his mugshot popped up, along with a giant green tick. Abdullah instantly pulled his finger away, in the hope that the result would change, but it was no use.

'There is a hundred per cent match,' the interrogator smiled, hoping the ruse had worked. 'We know you planted the bomb, Abdullah. If you confess, we might be able to go easy on you, but if you don't, then no big deal, because you'll be going to prison for a long time.' At this we all made a move to leave the room.

'Wait!' he shouted, standing up, now desperate. 'I have more information.'

Despite all his earlier bravado, when the going got tough he not only confessed but also snitched on his friends in an attempt to save himself, as so many of the people we brought in did. While the court did not accept the DNA analysis as evidence, as we had suspected, they did accept Abdullah's confession, and he was sentenced to life in jail. Such methods might not have been admissible in UK courts, but the Afghan legal system certainly had no issue with them. His evidence also enabled the arrest of other bomb makers and ensured they were also kept behind bars.

Everything had been moving so quickly that I didn't quite realize what a leap in capability I had just made. I haven't had very many good ideas in my life, but using the PCR machines to match human DNA in the field was definitely one of them. With the Afghan courts soon coming to accept DNA evidence, this new speeded-up process saw hundreds of Taliban fighters identified and convicted, especially after British soldiers visited villages and towns to take samples of DNA from every male of fighting age. As soon as there was an attack the authorities now had a better idea of who was responsible. Even if they didn't, when they did eventually bring a suspect into custody, they no longer had to wait fourteen days to test their DNA. The process was pretty much instantaneous.

I was ecstatic that my idea had enjoyed so much success. And the more I thought about it the more I felt that, if utilized properly, this could make a tremendous difference and possibly have great business potential. I just couldn't get the idea out of my head. The problem was, I didn't know where to start. I wasn't a businessman; I'd spent my entire life in the army.

However, even before I had this idea, as you may have already noticed, I had started to question my place in the military. After twenty-three years, I was becoming fed up with just being another staff officer. The invitation to sit the Higher Command and Staff Course was still pending and I had come to realize that maybe my character didn't really fit into the 'modern' army structure. I was too free and lateral of thought and would question things if they didn't make sense to me. Looking back on the supposed promotion to head up the CBRN team, I thought perhaps that had been a warning that my superiors felt the same way about me. While on the surface my annual reports seemed to be positive, describing me as a 'brilliant commanding officer', they also described me as a 'maverick'. Anyone who has been in the armed forces will tell you that the m-word is a slightly underhand way of saying that this man can't be trusted in the top positions. The way things had been going, I just couldn't see myself climbing the ladder, certainly not to where I wanted to go. And I had to admit, the buzz of being an army man had also started to wear off. I was growing increasingly restless, and the thought of going on tour no longer gave me the adrenalin rush that it once had. For the first time in my life I was probably guilty of going through the motions.

On my return home, with my frustration mounting, I told Julia that I was thinking of looking into another career. I think she was stunned. I was a military man through and through. The thought of me doing anything else seemed utterly ridiculous.

'Well, what would you do?' she asked.

'When I was in Afghanistan, I had an idea,' I replied, telling her about using the PCR machine to match human DNA in the field. 'I think there is a business opportunity there.'

While Julia was very supportive of me broadening my horizons, we needed to think through the finances carefully. We were lucky that the army had so far funded our children's schooling, through its Continuity of Education scheme, designed to provide some stability to the children of personnel and make up for the relatively meagre pay we received as soldiers. There was no way I was going to pull the children out of school, so anything I did decide to do had, as a minimum, to pay their fees, and they weren't cheap.

Indeed, I recognized that the grass wasn't always greener on the other side. Over the years, many of my brilliant colleagues had left the military to utilize their unique skills in the private sector. Fame and fortune apparently awaited but the reality was sometimes very different from what they expected. Many were unable to adapt, while some quickly ended up unemployed and severely depressed, regretting the day they ever left the loving embrace of the armed forces. I thought that perhaps what I was experiencing was just some sort of mid-life crisis that everyone in the military goes through. What I really needed to do was put all these thought out of my mind and knuckle back down.

However, just two weeks before I was due to fly back to Afghanistan, I attended Cheltenham Races with an old university friend, Andrew 'Duckie' Duckworth. Duckie was a very successful businessman, and when I happened to mention the PCR incident in Afghanistan, and my idea, he instantly grasped its potential. 'You need to commercialize it,' he urged. 'And my partners and I will back you!'

Despite all of my misgivings, I realized that this was a unique opportunity I would be foolish not to take. I had a chance to head up my own business, which could make a tremendous difference, backed by a very good friend. The money wouldn't be fantastic to begin with. I would have to earn my keep, but if Julia and I made some cutbacks, we could just about afford to keep paying the kids' school fees.

So, with a handshake, and a few pints to celebrate, I made up my mind to embark on a new career. Soon after, I handed in my notice to the military. There was no great goodbye or even any real thanks for my service. After serving a few months' notice, in September 2011, I merely handed over my military ID to some faceless civil servant in Andover and that was it: I was a civvie, and out in the wild. It was a scary feeling suddenly being cut loose, far scarier than any war zone I had encountered. After all the talk, it was time to sink or swim.

But far from offering a future sat comfortably behind a desk, this move would send me hurtling into some of the scariest war zones and chemical attacks ever perpetrated, starting with a trip to Kurdistan.

7

New Beginnings

Once I was out of the military, things moved pretty rapidly. Naming the company SecureBio, I managed to rent some office space at Porton Down. This really made it feel an integral part of the chemical community, plus it was a very cool address to put on our stationery. More importantly, it would allow us to mix with the world's best experts, get the most up-to-date data and equipment, and also ensure that we never lost sight of the fact that that while this was a business it could also have a major impact in the real world. But there was no way I could do this all alone.

First to join me was an old mate of mine, Ian 'Thommo' Thomson. Thommo was not only a fellow ex-Tankie, he had also been my Regimental Sergeant Major when I was CO of the CBRN Regiment. What this guy didn't know about chemical weapons wasn't worth knowing. He was truly a black belt on the subject. Since leaving the military, he had been operating on a consultancy basis to major organizations, but when I asked if he fancied getting involved with SecureBio, he jumped at the chance. While I knew his CBRN knowledge would prove to be invaluable, I also knew from experience that he would be great fun to work with, and that was certainly something I valued. There was no point to this if we weren't going to enjoy ourselves along the way.

Soon after, we were joined by Richie Mead, a former sergeant in the Metropolitan Police, who was also a CBRN expert. He knew the ins and outs of how to prevent and deal with home-soil chemical attacks, so having him on board would really cover our bases. Olly Morton, another ex-Tankie, also joined the ranks. Ready for life outside the military, Olly had retired early to seek a new challenge. Like me, he was surprised to find he had a real interest in CBRN and asked if he could come to us for some work experience. He fitted in so well, and was so keen to learn, that he soon became an integral part of the team.

Working alongside other ex-military men helped me to settle into my new role. We had all shared similar experiences, while we also had similar personalities and backgrounds. No matter our thoughts on the military, we all missed the camaraderie that it could bring. That day-to-day bond is something that is very difficult to replicate elsewhere. Thankfully, while these were now very different circumstances, the banter was soon flying, making the company feel like a mini regiment, ready to go to war for each other.

Good vibes were all well and good, but to stay afloat we desperately needed to attract some business, particularly as Julia had some bombshell news: she been made redundant. This was a huge blow, especially as my lump-sum gratuity from the army, which I had been relying on to see us through the first few lean months, was already dwindling away. If I hadn't been feeling the pressure to make ends meet before, I certainly was now. For a moment I wondered if I had bitten off more than I could chew and craved the warm embrace of military life and job security. But I knew that was in the past now. I had to look forward and somehow make this work, so for the first few weeks I was like a dog with a bone, tenaciously looking for work. I pumped all of my contacts for any leads, tossed my business card here, there and everywhere, and sent out hundreds of cold-call emails, hoping someone would bite. Eventually, they did.

One afternoon, as I portrayed to the guys the image of a duck swimming on water, all calm up above but paddling furiously down below, we suddenly received a phone call. No one had called for days, so as the phone rang all eyes were on me as I hastily grabbed the receiver.

'SecureBio,' I answered.

'Can I speak to Hamish, please?' came a male voice.

'Yes, Hamish speaking. How can I help you?'

'I'm from The International Commission for Missing

Persons. We received your email and have a project we might need your help with.'

At this, he proceeded to explain what he had in mind.

Following Saddam Hussein's gassing of the Kurds in 1988, thousands of contaminated bodies had been piled into a mass grave in Halabja. Due to the risk of cross contamination, it had been too dangerous to exhume the remains in order to identify the bodies. However, Secure-Bio could create a hot zone over the grave site, exhume the bodies and test their DNA against that of living family members in our PCR machines. There was now no need to transport thousands of contaminated bodies to a lab hundreds of miles away. We could do the procedure in Halabja itself.

It was just the type of project SecureBio was made for. Those families must have suffered tremendously in the years that had followed this attack and it gave me a great feeling of satisfaction that we could help. However, before we could do anything, I needed to get myself out to Halabja to inspect the site itself.

Flying into the Kurdish capital, Erbil, I wasn't quite sure what to expect. I suppose I had had in mind a crumbling, war-torn city, still trying to get back on its feet after the 2003 invasion of Iraq and decades of war. But from the moment I landed in the bustling new airport, it was clear that everything about this place was far from what I had envisioned. Having actually escaped the worst of the fighting in 2003, the city was unlike any other I had visited in Iraq. It was very modern and vibrant, almost like Dubai, with foreign investment helping to build glittering tower blocks. The city also welcomed thousands of tourists every year, and it was easy to see why. It boasted a warm climate all year round, and there was plenty to see and do, such as visit the World Heritage Site at the Citadel of Erbil, which overlooked the city from a huge mound, as well as the shops and restaurants at the Family Mall, and the incredible Bekhal and Gali Ali Bag natural waterfalls.

But I wasn't in Kurdistan to sightsee, not on this occasion anyway. I had work to do, so after a peaceful night in my hotel I was picked up by my driver and we set off for Halabja, which was around four hours away. With time to kill, my driver introduced himself as Afran and wanted to talk about Manchester United. He was a massive fan and seemed to know more than the average Brit. After peppering me with questions about Wayne Rooney and Old Trafford, he eventually came to ask my reason for visiting Halabja. When I told him, he shook his head.

'It is bad, you know, what has happened to us,' he said. 'We Kurds are proud people but it has not been easy.'

At this we delved into the Kurds' long quest for independence. While I knew some of the basics, picked up during my time in Iraq, I was certainly no expert on the subject, so it was interesting to hear Afran's thoughts.

The Kurds occupy parts of Turkey, Iraq, Syria, Iran and Armenia, and are united through race, culture and language but they don't have a state to call their own. This was, however, meant to change following the First World War, when Sir Mark Sykes and François Georges-Picot, the principal architects of the post-war world order, redrew many of the borders in the Middle East, with provision for a Kurdish state made in the 1920 Treaty of Sevres.

'Those bastards, Sykes and Picot,' Afran cursed. 'All of this is because of them.'

It was clear from the way Afran spat out the names of Sykes and Picot that things had not turned out as planned. Indeed, while the names of these two men might be long-forgotten by many in the West, in Kurdistan, and large parts of the Middle East, they are remembered and reviled for what is seen as the ultimate act of betrayal. Despite their many promises of independence, in 1923 the Treaty of Lausanne set the boundaries of modern Turkey and made no provision for a Kurdish state, leaving the Kurds with minority status in their respective countries. A raging sense of injustice erupted, which would mark the rest of the century and beyond.

In 1946, the Kurdistan Democratic Party (KDP) was formed to fight for autonomy in Iraq, culminating in the First Iraqi–Kurdish War (1961–70), which resulted in 100,000 casualties. Despite peace talks, promises were again broken, resulting in further conflict and bloodshed.

However, things reached another level with the rise of Saddam Hussein and the Iran–Iraq War in the 1980s. When the KDP backed the Islamic Republic, Saddam embarked on a series of vicious assaults to bring the Kurds to heel, including ordering his army to abduct as many as 8,000 men and boys from Erbil Province, who were imprisoned, tortured and murdered.

However, it was in the so-called Anfal campaign that the Kurds really felt the full force of Saddam's reprisals. Beginning in 1986, Iraqi forces sought to wipe the Kurds from the face of the earth, with ground offensives, aerial bombing, systematic destruction of settlements, mass deportation, firing squads and chemical warfare. It was during this campaign that Halabja was attacked.

Yet the Kurds survived these acts of genocide, and following Saddam's defeat in the Gulf War, they once again embarked on their bitter quest for independence. However, it wasn't until the Kurds helped US forces to oust Saddam in 2003 that they finally made some progress, as Jalal Talabani, a Kurd, replaced Saddam as President of Iraq. For now, at least in Iraq, the Kurds were reasonably happy with their lot, although it was clear from the way Afran spoke that Iraqis were still seen as the enemy, and not all the wounds were yet healed, especially those concerning Halabja.

As we continued talking, I was suddenly blown away by a scene of breathtaking beauty. Surrounded by snow-covered mountains on all sides, we turned a corner to see the bustling desert city of Sulaymaniyah, home to almost 700,000 people, shimmering below, looking like a jewel cupped in a giant pair of hands. I'd never seen anything quite so beautiful. Once more this extraordinary country took my breath away and shattered my preconceptions.

Within the hour we had arrived at our destination: Halabja. With a population of close to 250,000, this city, too, surprised me by its size and modernity. Upon my arrival I was greeted by the Mayor, as well as the Minister for Martyrs and Anfal Affairs. The Minister was a delightful man, who, I learnt, had been a Peshmerga fighter before escaping to the UK, through Iran, in the 1980s. He had taught at a London university for many years but had returned home after the fall of Saddam. We talked about the aftermath of the first Gulf War and he expressed his gratitude to the UK for setting up a no-fly zone over northern Iraq, to stop Saddam from targeting the Kurds and bombing them into oblivion.

'The two men I want to meet most are Sir John Major, who set up the NFZ,' he told me, 'and Tony Blair, who committed the British forces to defeat Saddam.'

'That's interesting,' I said with a smile. 'I think you might be in a small minority there, but I agree – I would like to meet them as well.'

Once we had exchanged polite pleasantries, our discussion soon turned to the reason for my visit.

'Please, come with us to see the museum and monument first,' the Minister pleaded. 'We think it is important.'

He was right. Arriving at the museum, on the outskirts of the city, I was immediately aware of the thousands of gravestones covering the landscape, going on for as far as the eye could see. 'They were all killed in the Anfal campaign by Saddam,' the Mayor said sorrowfully, as we both took a moment, trying to comprehend the enormity of this tragedy, all the pain and suffering, and the families that had been torn apart.

Soon after, I was presented to our guides, survivors of the actual attack, who told me what had happened on that awful day.

On the evening of 16 March 1988, the Iraqi Air Force dropped a series of bombs on Halabja. As this was during the height of the Anfal campaign, it was thought that these were conventional munitions. However, as the bombs hit the ground, they didn't explode as other bombs had done; instead clouds of white, black and yellow smoke billowed upwards, rising as a column about 150 feet in the air. This had certainly not been seen before.

As the cloud engulfed the streets, cries went out, 'Gas! Gas!' Panic ensued as people tried to escape, sprinting into buildings, jumping into cars, hiding in basements, but by and large it was useless. There was no escape. No matter where people hid, the gas could still seep through the cracks, so that the civilians had to inhale the noxious fumes that smelt of apples and eggs. Vomiting a green liquid, many gasped for breath, their skin breaking out in blisters, while others lost control of their limbs and bodily functions. Some died laughing. Men, women and children all succumbed. No one was immune to the death, or the terror. Whole families were wiped out in an instant.

A subsequent United Nations investigation concluded that mustard gas was used in the attack, along with nerve agents, such as tabun, sarin and VX.

'Do you know why Saddam used so many different nerve agents?' our guide asked me. I had no idea. 'It was to confuse the medics,' she replied. 'When thousands of casualties arrived at the hospital, many with different symptoms, they had no idea what they were dealing with. It made it impossible for the doctors to treat the victims until it was too late.'

If using nerve agents on civilians wasn't horrifying enough, this genuinely repulsed me. It takes a certain kind of wickedness to conjure up such a plan, that not even Adolf Hitler was guilty of.

Yet the pain of the Kurds was not at an end. Despite this attack happening over twenty years ago, many survivors were still being treated for the after-effects. Cancer was rife, as were miscarriages, still births and birth deformities. Perhaps most painful of all for many Kurds, Saddam got away with it. Though he had been put on trial for numerous war crimes in 2006, he was executed before he could be found guilty of this appalling crime, the likes of which had not, at that stage, been seen before.

It was a horrifying story, told very powerfully by its survivors. It brought tears to my eyes – not an easy thing to do. These people had all suffered so much, yet the world had not helped them. In fact, in many cases it had deceived and cheated them. My heart broke for all they had been through. I hoped that I might now be able to offer a semblance of peace.

Following this, we all set off to the scene of the attack, the old town of Halabja, which had barely changed, forever stuck in time: 16 March 1988. There, in the centre of this ghost town, was the mass grave that held the bodies of over 1,500 people, who had quickly been buried to avoid contaminating others. Though dealing with chemical weapons had been a part of my life for a few years by now, I was yet to see the end result. Standing by the grave, alongside those who had lost their loved ones, was a very moving experience. Below us were the bodies of thousands of innocent souls, who had died in the most horrific way; it was unimaginable. Now that a relative peace had fallen over Iraq, for the first time in decades, I promised my Kurdish friends that we would do all we could to help them.

Saying my goodbyes to my new friends in Halabja, I was proud that this would be SecureBio's first job. It would, however, take some months to prepare the operation. In the meantime, I came up with another idea that we could add to our services, as well as help our cash flow. Following the 2001 anthrax attack on the US Postal Service, there had been a further 69,000 reported white powder attacks, almost all of which were fake. One of the most prolific hoaxers was Clayton Waagner, an anti-abortion activist, who mailed hundreds of anthrax hoax letters to abortion clinics in America.

However, most of these fake attacks targeted high-profile or powerful individuals, such as politicians and bankers. Though the attacks were fake, they still caused chaos. Buildings had to be evacuated, costing millions of pounds in lost business, and anyone who thought they might have come into contact with anthrax had to be rushed to hospital.

With all this in mind, we created a mobile biological detection system, which could test any such powder as soon as an envelope was opened. If the powder was found to be harmless, this would negate the need to evacuate the building or send anyone to hospital. For banks this was especially important. Closing their office for a day could cost upwards of tens of millions of pounds. Unsurprisingly, companies such as Goldman Sachs were particularly inter-ested in the service.

While the business seemed to have made a solid start, and for now I had put our money worries to bed, I still felt the urge for something more. I had been well aware that I would miss the adrenalin rush of being in a war zone, and I was somewhat prepared for this, but my competitive instincts were still hard to quell. I needed a purpose or an element of excitement to really give me what I craved. Hearing this, Julia suggested I enter the London Marathon. It was a suggestion that would almost kill me.

8

Sudden Death

My heart suddenly clenched tight. My head started to swirl and my legs buckled. Staggering to the floor. I tried to catch my breath. But each breath was agony. *I can't be having a heart attack*, I thought. *I'm only forty-eight and the fittest I've ever been.*

Over the previous few weeks, I had been training for the London Marathon with a series of personal bests. I was flying. Every morning before work I pounded the pavements around Salisbury, increasing my mileage and improving my time. I relished the challenge and was soon reaching levels of fitness I hadn't been at since my early twenties. It also gave me an escape from my desk and got the blood pumping, especially as I was hoping to raise money for charity. I felt pretty good about myself, and about life. Things looked to be working out OK. But then one morning, as I pushed myself harder and harder, legs pumping, heart pounding, everything suddenly went black.

Seconds later I was flat on my back starring at the sky, wondering: *Is this it?*

After being checked out at the local hospital, I was rushed to the London Chest Hospital, where I was examined by Professor Perry Elliot.

'I feel fine now,' I told him. 'I probably didn't eat enough before I went running.'

Deep down, I knew this was a lie. I knew all too well what exercising on an empty stomach and feeling faint as a result felt like, and this was nothing like that. It had felt like the world was spinning down a drain and sucking me down with it, swirling and swirling until there was total darkness. It had been a pretty scary experience but I certainly didn't want to admit this might be something serious.

Again, my time at boarding school and in the military meant that I was still pretty old school when it came to injuries and illness. I was like that famous Monty Python sketch when the knight keeps getting body parts chopped off: 'Just a scratch, old chap.' I can't actually remember ever feeling ill, or certainly not ill enough to take a day off school or work. When I played rugby, I sustained some pretty nasty injuries, but I had always got back up and played on, again not wanting to show any weakness. Besides, I really was feeling back to my old self. I had only gone to the hospital because Julia had practically forced me. The last thing I wanted to hear right now was that I had some sort of health issue, particularly when I had a marathon to train for.

'We'll soon see what's really going on, Colonel,' the professor promised, handing me a heart monitor.

At this, he asked me to jog on a running machine while he monitored my readings. Never one for half measures, I was soon pounding the treadmill, going faster and faster, feeling pretty damn good actually. *If I was ill, could I really be running flat out like this?* I thought, wanting to show myself, and the doctor, that I was in peak physical fitness.

'Stop! Stop!' the professor suddenly cried, urging me to step off the machine.

I thought he had seen enough, that my readings had been so good that there was no need to continue. But it was quite the opposite.

'How did you feel just then?' he asked, still looking at my readings with an air of concern.

'I felt great,' I said. 'Nothing like before.'

The professor raised his eyebrows and looked back at my readings.

'Judging by this, you were on the verge of having a heart attack,' he said. 'Your heart had actually gone into spasm.'

This shocked me. I had not felt a thing. I had felt as fit and healthy as I had ever been. In fact, I had just been about to push myself even harder. None of this made any sense. Surely there was some sort of mistake? How could

I have been on the verge of having a heart attack and not felt a thing?

After further tests by cardiologists, including an echocardiogram so they could see my heart beating in real time, I was hit with the bad news: 'I'm afraid you have hypertrophic cardiomyopathy.' This meant nothing to me but when I was told it was otherwise known as 'sudden cardiac death syndrome', I soon realized it was pretty damn serious.

Apparently, I had a thickening of the heart muscle that could cause sudden death if I was subjected to too much stress. That made me laugh. Having served in Afghanistan and Iraq, I was astonished that I had survived this long. In fact, I was extremely lucky to have the condition diagnosed before it was too late – 90% of sufferers are dead before they get that chance. Unsurprisingly, it was recommended that I take it easy from here on in. It appeared that going to war zones was definitely out of the question.

'Thank God you decided to get out of the military when you did,' Julia said, tending to me as if I was a poorly patient. But I tried not to make a big thing of it. Once again, on the surface, I was all bravado. I claimed that some of the world's worst war zones hadn't got me yet so a dicky heart certainly wasn't going to put an end to me. However, I must admit, I was scared. My unshakeable self-confidence had been well and truly rattled. I felt like I had a ticking time bomb in my chest that could explode at any moment. If the tests had shown I was on the verge of a heart attack and I hadn't felt a thing, then I would have no indication of when this thing was going to strike. It was a bloody miracle my heart hadn't already exploded during some of the scrapes I had got myself into over the years.

For a number of days, I barely moved, unsure of what my body was now capable of. Just breaking into anything more than a walk set my mind racing. *Is this it? Is that funny feeling my heart about to go?* Every morning I would go for a short stroll, gradually building my confidence, but this didn't last for long. I had no interest in walking. I wanted to run. To really push myself and ignore the consequences, but I had to follow doctors' orders. I had to be sensible. But, as I said to Julia when she quoted this back to me: 'When have I ever been sensible!?'

Soon I was climbing the walls. I felt old, as if my best days were now firmly behind me. I had always prided myself on my physical fitness, taking it as an affront if anyone should beat me at any exercise. Now even walking around the house had me worried. I was meant to be a military man. The one-time world press-up champion no less! My self-image had been shattered. Still, I consoled myself that at least I had made the decision to quit the army before that decision had been made for me. There was no way I would have been able to serve with this hanging over me. It would have been extremely distressing to be relieved of duty, with no plans in place.

I became increasingly angry, snapping at anyone at home or at work, for just about anything. Any minor digression was leapt upon, and the worst thing anyone could say to me was: How are you feeling? This was like a red rag to a bull. *Mind your bloody business,* I wanted to shout back. Everything just felt wet and grey. I didn't know how to process it all but I knew one thing for certain: this was no way to live. I had to find a way to get back to some semblance of normality. I needed the buzz!

I was told that beta blockers might be the solution I was looking for. These tablets would apparently restrict my heart rate to just 140 beats per minute, down from around 200. This would decrease the risk of having a heart attack, although I was warned that it was no guarantee. If I was subjected to too much stress, there was no telling how my heart would react. Everyone reacted differently to this condition. You just had to be careful. *Forget about that.* I refused to live my life in fear. If it got me, then it got me. I intended to live my life to the full.

So, knocking back beta blockers, I told Julia I was going to do some shopping but instead went to my local gym. It was like a covert operation. I knew that if anyone who knew about my condition should see me, they would try to talk me out of it. But this was something I just had to do. Others couldn't understand why I would want to put myself in any danger but, right or wrong, that has always been a key part of my make-up.

After a reconnaissance of the gym, to check there was no one around who might know me, I hit the running machine. Soon I was in my stride, minute by minute upping the pace. I felt good. Really good, in fact. As if there was nothing wrong at all. But suddenly my legs started to feel heavy, as if my feet had been plunged into concrete. I tried to take a deep breath, and power through, but there was no more room in my lungs. It was as if a child had jumped on my back and was trying to drag me down. Soon I had to stop, puffing and panting, down on all fours, drenched in sweat. I must have looked a right state, but it wasn't a heart attack I was having, it was the bloody beta blockers. My doctor had warned me about this. With my heart rate restricted, I no longer had anything like the capacity I'd had previously.

I found this tremendously frustrating. When Julia had finished scolding me, after she found I had been to the gym, she told me I was lucky to be able to exercise at all. I knew this, but that competitive instinct refused to go away. *You can do this, Hamish,* my mind continually urged, but it seemed no matter how hard I pushed I would keep hitting a brick wall.

That was when one of Britain's greatest ever athletes, Mo Farah, saved me – even though he won't know it, as we've never met. One day I read that when he hits top speed his heart rate is only around 140 beats a minute. This was, of course, the same heart rate as mine with the beta blockers. So, if Mo Farah could break world records with such a heart rate, what was my excuse?

I became obsessed with studying Mo, and other endurance athletes, to see how they trained. What was their secret? The more I read the more I found that little changes could make all the difference. I adjusted my gait, looking to run more efficiently, having learnt that Farah keeps his hips and shoulders level, while his legs move straight forward, meaning there is no unnecessary side-to-side movement or twisting. I also studied foot positioning, noticing that many amateur runners, like myself, strike the ground first with their heels, which causes a large impact force to run up their legs to their knees and hips. Farah, however, strikes the ground with the ball of his foot, and then lowers his heel before going back up on to the ball of his foot and pushing away with his toes, essentially becoming lighter on his feet. All this ensured an optimal range of movement, increasing speed while decreasing effort.

Perhaps the biggest game-changer was watching YouTube videos on how to breathe properly. It sounds ridiculous but there's a real art to breathing when running, which ensures you get far more bang for your buck. Respiration is, of course, a chemical process. Put very simply, we breathe in oxygen and breathe out carbon dioxide. I just needed to find a way to make my lungs more efficient so I could breathe in more oxygen and breathe out more carbon dioxide.

I learnt that a major mistake a lot of sports people make is breathing from their chest instead of their diaphragm, as this limits oxygen intake. So I tried 'belly breaths', placing my hand on my stomach, taking slow, deep breaths, lifting my hand as I inhaled and sinking it as I exhaled, until this became a natural thing to do. From there, I focused on inhaling deeply through my nose, again taking in more oxygen, and out through my mouth, releasing more carbon dioxide. While this helped make my breathing far more efficient, what made a real difference was using this method for rhythmic breathing, inhaling for two counts, then exhaling for two counts. Suddenly my lung capacity felt much larger; I was taking in far more oxygen and releasing far more carbon dioxide, ensuring a steady flow of oxygen to my muscles.

All of these little changes, as well as a few others, had a big impact. While I was not yet at my previous level of fitness, I could feel myself improving and breaking through the beta blocker-imposed brick wall. It's somewhat ironic that studying the chemical reactions of breathing proved to be so crucial. I had once run from all talk of chemicals, now they had changed my life, in more ways than one.

Feeling more like myself, and gaining confidence, I made it my goal to push myself to see if I could still pass the army's fitness test for new recruits. This entailed running 1.5 miles in under 11.5 minutes and then another 1.5 miles in under 10.5 minutes. Normally this would have been a piece of cake, but I didn't just want to pass the test, I wanted to annihilate it, to get back to where I had been. I think when I had first passed the test I had finished the first 1.5 miles in 10 minutes and the second in 9.5 minutes. This was therefore my goal.

But one night I heard Julia shout from downstairs, 'Hamish! Quick! Turn on the news!' Turning the TV on, I saw a breaking news story that the Bolton Wanderers footballer Fabrice Muamba had suffered a cardiac arrest during a game against Tottenham Hotspur. One minute he had been jogging in the middle of the pitch, the next he had fallen like a tree, as if the lights had suddenly been switched out. Medics raced to help and found his heart had stopped beating. He was given a defibrillator shock on the pitch, then he was rushed to the London Chest Hospital, where he was now in intensive care. In the days that followed, he thankfully recovered but was soon diagnosed with sudden cardiac death syndrome. Sadly, at twenty-three years of age, his football career was over, but I imagine he was just glad to be alive.

Watching footage of a young man, in the prime of his life, collapse and almost die, with a similar condition to the one I had, knocked me for six. If it wasn't for the fact he'd been in a football stadium and surrounded by medics, and medical equipment, then he would have surely died. If the same should ever happen to me, then, like most others, I would not be so lucky. For a few days I wondered if I should just quit while I was ahead. If a young man like Fabrice Muamba had to come to terms with his career being over, what made me so special? Why did I have to put myself, and my family, through all of this worry when I could just sit back and look after myself?

Of course, my mind got the better of me. *Normal life is boring . . . You've trained hard . . . You're taking beta blockers . . . You're looking for a way out . . . You're just cheating yourself!* I knew that these thoughts would not rest until I had completed the test.

The next morning, I decided not to torture myself any longer. Come what may, today was the day. I went into the countryside at the break of dawn, with a stop watch in my hand and my pet Labrador, Butler, running loyally alongside me. Having taken the beta blockers, I set off, giving it all I had. It was almost as if I was testing whether I was still the same person. My identity had always been entwined with my physical fitness, and in being one of the fittest in the army. If, at forty-eight, I could no longer get anywhere near my previous time or if I could not complete the test at all, I would have found this very challenging.

As I came up to the first 1.5 miles I looked down at the watch in my hand: 10 minutes and 25 seconds. I had completed the first part well under time! I felt elated, but the hard work would come in the second 1.5 miles. This was when the legs would bite, the lungs would burn and the beta blockers would really kick in. Gritting my teeth, I told myself: *Two breaths in . . . two breaths out . . .* like a mantra, taking in the air through my nose, breathing out through my mouth, watching the carbon dioxide turn to mist in the early morning cold. Actually, seeing my breath only helped me regulate my breathing more efficiently, as did Butler running up ahead, acting as a pacemaker. Checking the stopwatch, I realized I was close to the time I had set as young recruit. At this my feet picked up . . . the end in sight . . . deeper and deeper breaths . . . my legs getting heavy and heavier . . . the finish line getting closer . . .

Racing across, I pressed stop on the watch and hunched over, panting and wheezing, Butler licking my face, glancing down at my time: 9 minutes and 55 seconds. *Bloody hell!* I wasn't far off the time I had set as a twenty-one-year-old. I couldn't believe it. I felt like punching the air like Rocky and roaring out, 'Adrian!' Instead, I hugged Butler and let out a guttural scream. Even now, at forty-eight years of age, with a dicky heart and on beta blockers, I could still pass the army fitness test with flying colours. And best of all, I felt great – better than ever, in fact, as if nothing had ever happened. I knew there was a danger of complacency, that I could be feeling fine and then suddenly drop dead, but I couldn't live my life with that thought hanging over me. I had managed to adapt to my condition, and had become far more efficient in the process.

However, just as I felt I was making real progress with my health, the Middle East was again being torn apart by war. Once more, like a moth to a flame, heart condition or not, I felt the urge to get involved. And I would soon get my chance.

Part Two

'Like a Man in Fire'

9

The Arab Spring

It took the seemingly inconsequential assassination of Archduke Franz Ferdinand in 1914 to start the First World War. Similarly, it would also take a relatively unremarkable event in Tunisia to spark uprisings throughout North Africa, the Middle East and beyond, in a series of conflicts that would become known as the Arab Spring.

The spark was lit on the morning of 17 December 2010, in the Tunisian city of Sidi Bouzid. In the early hours, street vendor Tarek el-Tayeb Mohamed Bouazizi arrived at his patch, checked to see if the coast was clear, then set out produce to sell in a wheelbarrow. For a while now, life had been a struggle for Bouazizi, and his profession was on a knife edge. He had had to borrow money to buy this produce, and he was also being harassed by the police. It seemed that wherever he set up shop they suddenly turned up and demanded a bribe. If he could not pay them, his produce was confiscated and he would return home penniless. And Bouazizi could never afford to pay it. All of his money went on buying produce and feeding his family. If he were to pay the police as well, he would be left with nothing. So, every day, he had to change locations, quickly setting up shop, hoping to sell enough to pay back his loan and feed his family with the rest, all without being spotted by the police.

However, on this day, Bouazizi's luck was out again. At around 10.30 a.m., police officers arrived at the scene and once more accused him of not having a vendor's permit. Bouazizi knew the drill by now. While he explained that no such permit was required to sell from a cart, he knew his excuses would not matter. The only permit the police were interested in was cold hard cash. With no money, and no intention of handing over a penny, he once again refused to pay them.

Upon his refusal, Bouazizi was slapped in the face and spat on by a female municipal officer. He was then beaten and his scales and produce confiscated. Bloodied and humiliated, the angry Bouazizi snapped. Limping to the governor's office, he tried to lodge a complaint about the corrupt police. Yet no one was willing to listen to a man so low on the social scale, certainly not a man without funds to make people listen. So Bouazizi took the only action he believed was left for a man in his position. Less than an hour after the altercation he set himself on fire in the middle of a busy street. Three weeks later, he died from his injuries.

The Arab Spring

Outraged by these events, people took to the streets and protests soon spread throughout the country like wildfire. On 14 January 2011, with events spiralling out of control, President Ben Ali fled Tunisia with his family, ending his twenty-three-year rule. Inspired by these events, further uprisings erupted across the Middle East and North Africa. In Egypt, President Mubarak was toppled after thirty years in power, while Libyan President Colonel Gaddafi was dragged out of hiding and killed in the street. This was the biggest transformation of the Middle East since decolonization, and while many of the power struggles of the Arab Spring were all but over by the end of 2012, one such conflict was only just beginning.

For years, the people of Syria had been complaining about high unemployment, corruption, human rights violations and a lack of political freedom under the rule of President Bashar al-Assad. But with the Arab Spring exploding throughout the Middle East, the dissent that had been bubbling under the surface now rose to the top.

On 6 March 2011 matters came to a head, when children in the southern Syrian city of Daraa graffitied walls with anti-government messages. They were subsequently arrested and assaulted by the police. In response, thousands of protestors gathered throughout the country, including over 100,000 at the central square of Homs. With the government desperately trying to cling to power, army tanks stormed several cities on President Assad's orders, killing hundreds of protestors in the process. Opposition supporters subsequently took up arms to defend themselves, calling themselves the Free Syrian Army (FSA). The genie was now out of the bottle, as the violence escalated into a bloody civil war.

However, the Syrian conflict became far more complicated than other Arab Spring movements. Rather than just an anti-government group against a pro-government group, support was fractured along religious lines, with the Sunni Muslim majority set against the president's Shia Alawite sect. This allowed jihadist groups such as al-Qaeda, and later ISIS, to flourish, as both sought to gain advantage from the chaos and take over Syria, and Iraq, to form a Muslim caliphate.

Complicating matters further, other countries became embroiled in the conflict. With Russia and Iran supporting Assad, the likes of Turkey, the UK, USA and other Gulf Arab states backed the opposition. While this was complex in itself, many of the anti-Assad forces were also infiltrated by terror groups, which the UK and USA inadvertently found themselves supporting. As such, they could not risk providing the likes of the FSA with aid for fear it would fall into the wrong hands.

However, though the UK and USA had no intention of supporting terrorist groups, and might have sat back and allowed Assad and Putin to annihilate them, everyone was horrified at the lengths Assad's regime went to. In order to avoid capture, terrorists often hid in civilian populations, with Assad claiming they had a particular liking for hospitals and playgrounds. Yet Assad and Putin had no qualms about dropping bombs on such places if it meant a few of their enemies would be killed. As a result, thousands of innocents died in the process. But Assad had other, far more lethal – and effective – weapons at his disposal, which he was desperate to unleash.

According to US intelligence reports, Syria had begun to develop its chemical weapons capabilities in the late 1970s, thanks to supplies and training from the Soviet Union. By the late 1980s its chemical weapons programme was believed to be even more advanced than Iraq's, which is really saying something. As Syria was not a signatory to the Chemical Weapons Convention, Assad's regime was free to continue to develop and produce as many chemical weapons as it liked, culminating in what many believed to be the third largest chemical stockpile in the world, behind the United States and Russia. When war broke out, it was only a matter of time before Assad looked to use them.

Initially, such attacks on rebel forces were relatively 'small' scale, with the regime accused of using grenades full of sarin. While Assad was not bound by the Chemical Weapons Convention, he was still well aware that chemical attacks would not be taken lightly by the West. With these initial grenade attacks, it was almost as if he was testing the water to see if there would be any response. When none was forthcoming, the attacks became more widespread, and more deadly.

The real game-changer came on 19 March 2013, when in the early hours of the morning an object filled with sarin was dropped on to Khan al-Assal, a district of Aleppo. This resulted in at least twenty-six fatalities and more than eighty-six injuries, including to some of the medics who treated the victims at University Hospital in Aleppo.

At this point I was approached by the media to provide an expert opinion on the use of chemical weapons in Syria, appearing on such programmes as BBC Radio 4's *Today*. Invited to share my views on the matter, I certainly didn't pull any punches. Having recently seen just how horrific the situation had been in Halabja, I said that these actions in Syria urgently needing investigating and robust action must be taken if Assad was found to be guilty of such a war crime. As my name became more widely known in media circles, I was asked by the American TV network CBS to help their news team prepare for a trip into Syria itself. I had actually never been to Syria, but they wanted me to advise on the chemical weapons aspect, what equipment they would need, what to look out for and how to treat any injuries. However, as events in the Middle East intensified, the BBC soon had a different proposition altogether.

On 29 April 2013, shortly after midday, a helicopter was seen to be dropping objects on to Saraqeb, a rebel-held city in northwestern Syria. Shortly after, casualties began to arrive at the local hospital, with symptoms such as convulsions, frothing at the mouth, and pinpoint pupils. One of the victims, Mariam Khatib, was subsequently sent to a hospital in Turkey to be treated but died soon after. The attack and the symptoms again bore all the hallmarks of sarin.

Hearing that a nerve agent such as sarin might have been used on civilians appalled me. I had already seen the effect of such an attack on the Kurds in Halabja. Thousands had died and more than twenty years later people were still physically and psychologically haunted by it. While the casualties in Saraqeb did not yet appear to be anywhere near those levels, it was clear that this was the tip of the iceberg. If Assad wasn't stopped, things could escalate rapidly.

However, as Syria was not a signatory to the Chemical Weapons Convention, the country was not obligated to allow the UN's investigatory arm, the Organization for the Prohibition of Chemical Weapons (OPCW), in to investigate. This made it very difficult for the world to know what was truly going on and to take appropriate action. But that was about to change.

Soon after the attack, I received a call from Ian Pannell, the BBC's Middle East correspondent. 'I'm going to Saraqeb to report on the attacks,' he said. 'Would you be able to meet me at the Turkish border to review what I find?' I wasn't quite sure why I had to be at the border itself, and couldn't just do that from the UK, but I reasoned it probably made better TV if I was actually out there with Ian.

In any event, I didn't question the reasons. Despite my health issues, and though I was now running a business full-time, it was an opportunity I was keen to take. I reasoned that I wouldn't be away for no more than a few days, and as I would be on the border I would be out of harm's way. Also, I could help provide the BBC with some expert analysis on the attack and hopefully shine a light on to Assad's activities. In those circumstances there was nothing to worry about. I would be back at my desk in no time at all.

And so, in early May 2013, with my beta blockers packed, I said my goodbyes to my family, boarded a flight at Heathrow and made my way to Hatay, at the Turkish/ Syrian border. There, as promised, I was met by Ian Pannell and his team, who had just returned from Saraqeb.

Over the last few days, they had performed some extraordinary work, visiting the site of the attack, speaking to witnesses, doctors and even victims. The footage and photographs they had obtained were compelling. First-hand video footage showed the moment helicopters dropped the bombs on to a road in a suburban area, where black smoke dispersed on impact. Footage also showed victims arriving at the hospital, their eyes closed, heads tilted back, gasping for air, vomiting, while holding their heads in agony. Perhaps the most painful footage was that of Mariam Khatib's son, who relived the moment his mother had died after being transferred to Turkey. It was harrowing to watch, and it was clear to me that sarin had been used, as I outlined during my subsequent interview with Ian.

By this stage the President of the United States, Barack Obama, had already stated in reference to proposed military action against Assad: 'We have been very clear to the Assad regime, but also to other players on the ground, that a red line for us is if we start seeing a whole bunch of chemical weapons moving around or being utilized. That would change my calculus. That would change my equation.' It seemed to me that that 'red line' had been crossed and action now needed to be taken. However, without definite proof, no one was yet ready to pull the trigger.

As we travelled back to our hotel that night, I couldn't get the images of Saraqeb out of my head. It was clear that these sorts of atrocities were not going to stop, and if something wasn't done soon then we might very well have another Halabja on our hands. But OPCW inspectors could not get into Syria to investigate, no matter how great the global outcry. It appeared the matter was just going to be left alone. This was a thoroughly depressing thought, and one which drove me to the hotel bar for a drink. It was a decision which was to have far-reaching consequences.

10

The First Attempt

Entering the hotel bar shortly after 9.30 p.m., I found it virtually empty, which suited me down to the ground. I needed some solitude in order to run everything over in my head. It had been a very sobering experience watching all of the footage that Ian had taken and then realizing that it was unlikely that anything would be done. With this in mind, I ordered a bottle of red wine, fully intending to polish off the lot in the hope it would at least help me get to sleep.

As I worked my way through the bottle, minding my own business, I noticed a middle-aged man with greying hair walk into the bar. Ordering a drink, he proceeded to sit at the table opposite mine, which I found slightly unnerving, as the room was empty bar one or two fellow stragglers. Avoiding eye contact, I decided to finish off the remains of the bottle and make a move.

'How's it going?' the man suddenly asked, in an accent I couldn't quite place.

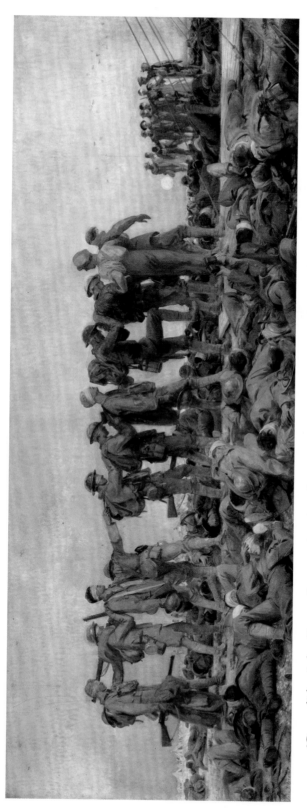

'Gassed' by John Singer Sargent (1919), depicting soldiers wounded by mustard gas in the First World War.

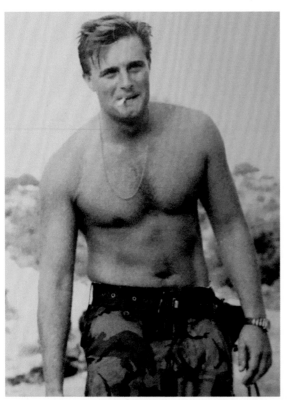

Left. As a young soldier on United Nations duty in Cyprus, 1989.

Below. My first tour in the Gulf.

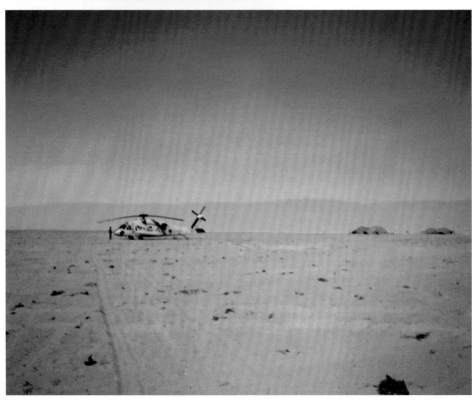

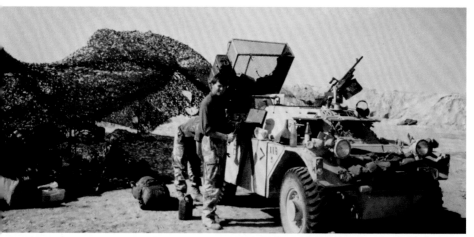

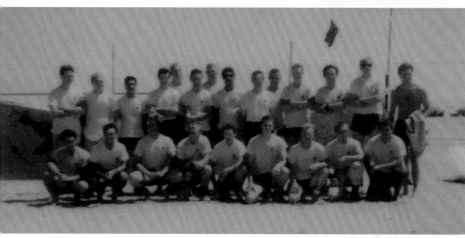

Top. First Gulf War preparing for battle somewhere in Saudi Arabia, Jan 1991.

Above. The Press-Up World Record attempt in the Kuwait desert, April 1991.

Right. A proud young tankie – Officer Commanding G Squadron 1RTR, Canada, 1997.

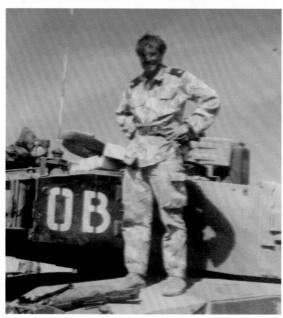

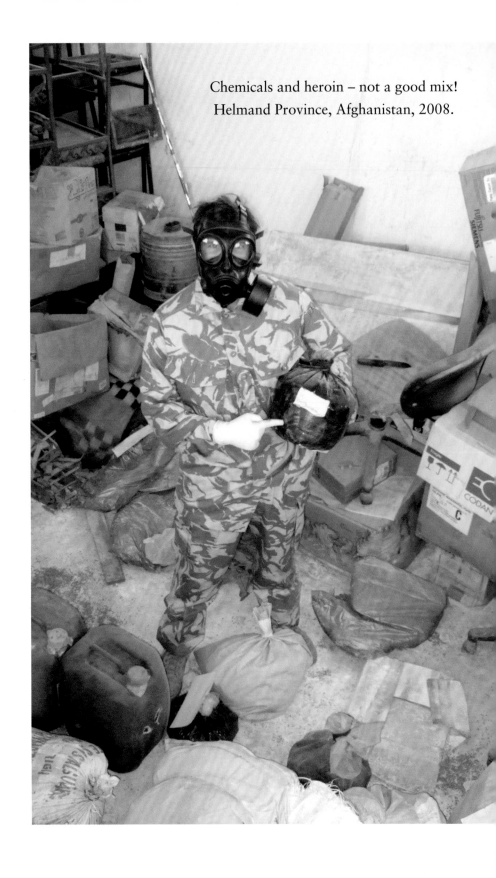

Chemicals and heroin – not a good mix!
Helmand Province, Afghanistan, 2008.

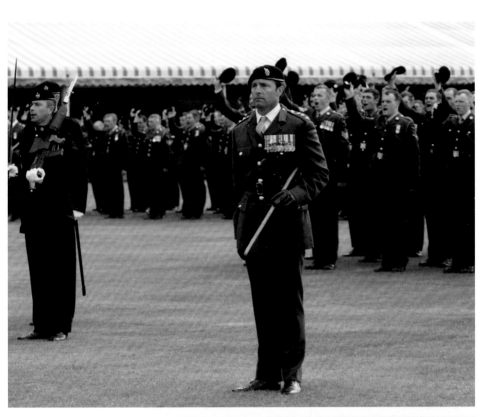

Above. Leading the Queen's RTR Standards Parade in 2008, just three years before leaving the army.

Right. Visiting the Peshmerga near Mosul, 2016.

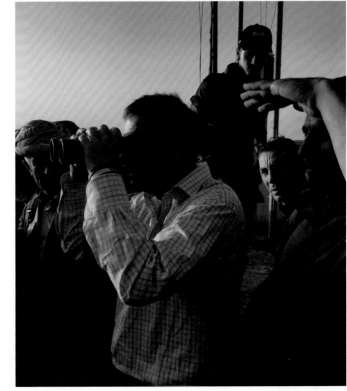

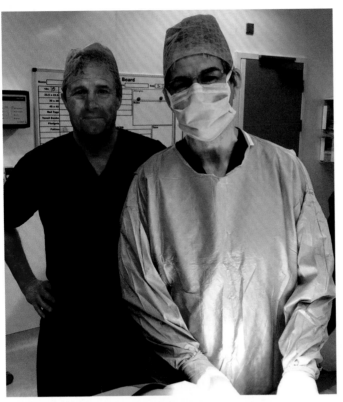

With my friend
David Nott,
in surgery (*left*)
and in Syria (*below*)
and also with
Dr Mounir,
July 2019.

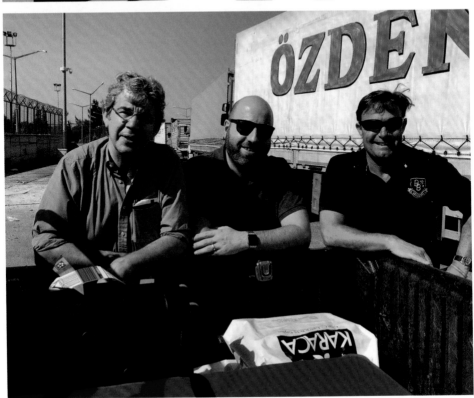

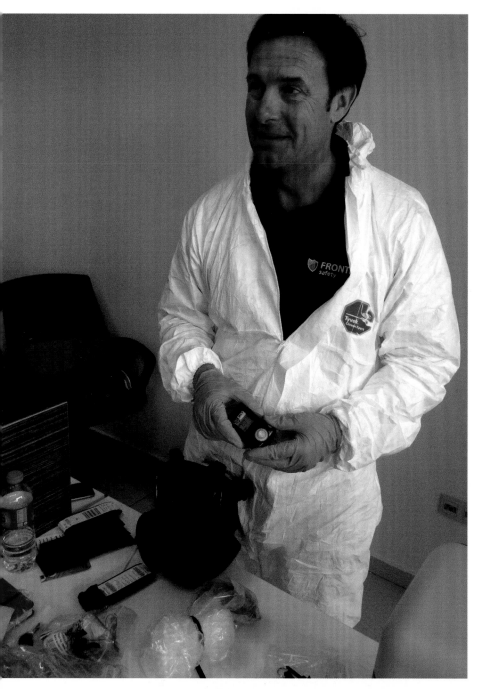

Collecting evidence at Bab Al Hawa Hospital in Syria.

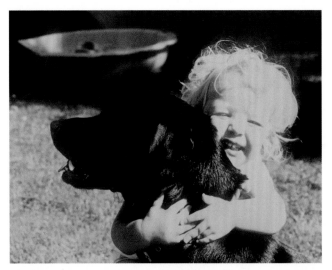

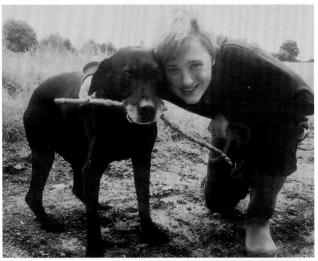

Jemima and Felix
with Butler the Dog.

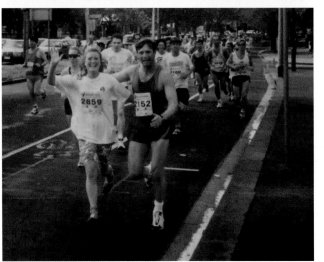

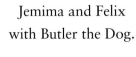

Running the
Melbourne marathon
with my wife, Julia.

'Good,' I replied, unsure where this was heading, but thinking that he seemed friendly enough.

Quickly, we rolled through the obligatory pleasantries. I learnt that his name was Hassan and that he was a Syrian, clearly wealthy, who had spent a lot of time in the West and was heading up a humanitarian mission to help impoverished villages in the Syrian province of Idlib. He seemed to know the area and the people very well, reeling off stories of others in the province he was in contact with, lawyers, doctors, politicians. He seemed to know everyone.

It was interesting to get an insider's perspective on the situation in Syria but while I was more than happy to let Hassan talk, I continued to keep my cards relatively close to my chest. At first, all I revealed was that I was British and that I was there on business. But as we continued to talk, and I realized Hassan was no danger and was just looking for casual conversation, as so many do late at night in hotel bars, I eventually told him that I was ex-military and was out here assisting the BBC, reporting on Saraqeb.

'That is a terrible business,' Hassan muttered, shaking his head. 'I have a friend who lives there. I told him he has to leave, this is just the beginning, but it is his home. Where is he to go?'

I shook my head in sympathy. This was an issue that would soon face so many of the Syrian people, and there was no real answer. The refugee crisis was just beginning, and with cities like Saraqeb on Assad's radar, I didn't see much hope for Hassan's friend unless he left quickly.

After half an hour of trading tidbits of information, and learning that Hassan was set to visit Idlib to deliver food and medicines the next day, I thanked him for his company and said goodnight. It had been good to talk, even if we had returned to the ever-depressing topic of the future of his homeland.

Returning to my room, I set my alarm for 6 a.m. and tried to get some sleep, but it was impossible.

As I lay awake, thinking everything over, a mad plan began to hatch in my head. With Hassan's help, I could go into Syria and collect samples from Saraqeb, take them back across the border and hand them to OPCW inspectors. The OPCW might not be permitted to enter the country but there was nothing stopping me. I was just a regular citizen, and by all accounts I wouldn't be breaking any laws, none that I was too concerned about anyway. It seemed to be the solution to so many problems. On the other hand, there was a long list of sensible reasons for me not to take such a risk. Indeed, I could almost hear the howls of protest from my family, business partners and doctors:

'You've been out of the army for two years and you're approaching middle age.'

'You have a serious health condition – any stress could kill you!'

150

'Do you realize there's a civil war going on in Syria and you'll be all alone?'

'The business is at a delicate stage; we can't afford to lose you.'

'It won't be the chemicals that will kill you but your own stupidity!'

I understood all of these concerns. Truly, I did. Syria looked like a hellhole. Any normal person would have run a million miles from the place. Every day there seemed to be another story of yet another atrocity, with rebels, terrorists and government forces running amok. But while these reasons not to go were all well and good, an overwhelming one to do so remained: I had to collect the samples to prove Assad was guilty. The OPCW couldn't do it, and it didn't look like anyone else was going to either. I knew this was vitally important, perhaps the most important thing I had ever done in my life. In the past, I had gone to war zones because it was my job. I had had no choice in the matter. Often, I hadn't really understood what we were doing in such places, nor had I cared. I had just wanted to get my boots on the ground. This time, though, I knew the stakes, and what would happen if action wasn't taken. This had all the hallmarks of another Halabja in the making, or worse. Something had to be done. A fire had been lit and I couldn't put it out.

While this was the primary thought in my head, looking back I understand now that there might have been more to it. Although I had more or less battled my way back to full health after my heart attack scare, I still felt I had something to prove to myself. Passing the new recruit army fitness test was one thing, but could I still operate in a volatile war zone? Maybe I wanted to prove to myself, and to others, that I wasn't ready for the knacker's yard just yet. I was also probably looking forward to once more tasting the chaos and mayhem of a war zone, which had always been like a drug to me. I appreciate that this sounds crazy to a sane person, but having spent my whole adult life living on the edge, I found it very difficult to adjust back to normality. I suppose I am easily bored, which is what Julia tells me she is going to put on my gravestone when I do eventually snuff it.

Before I could put any plans into action, I first had to speak to Hassan. But not knowing his second name, or even his room number, I had no way to contact him. All I could do was stake out the lobby in the hope of catching him before he departed. There was no time to waste. I had no idea when he was set to leave, so at 5.30 a.m. I made my way downstairs, watching everyone who crossed my path, hoping that he had not yet left. Then, just over an hour later, he emerged from the elevator.

'Hello, my friend,' he smiled, on seeing me. 'What are you doing here?'

'I have an idea,' I said. 'And I need your help.'

I explained my plan to Hassan. I would travel into Syria with him, as part of his aid convoy, and we would go to Saraqeb, collect the samples and bring them across the border to give to the OPCW. But there was a problem.

'It is too risky for you to go to Saraqeb,' he warned.

'The BBC news crew I have been working with have been there just recently,' I replied.

'Yes, but they were not taking samples from the site of the attack. If anyone sees a Westerner do this, it will be clear what you are doing. You will be killed.'

This was a good point. In my haste to get to Saraqeb, I had not thought of this.

'Listen,' Hassan said, the gears working in his head, 'I will call my friend Abdullah, in Saraqeb. Maybe he can collect the samples and meet us here, in Hatay.'

This sounded even better but first I needed to speak to Abdullah, and ensure he knew what to do, that is, if he even wanted to go along with all of this. Taking out his phone, Hassan made the call, and after he had explained everything, it was clear Abdullah was desperate to do all that he could to help us. As with many others, he would do absolutely anything to ensure the world knew of Assad's atrocities. But there was one issue: Abdullah did not want to risk taking the samples across the border into Turkey, fearing what would happen if he were caught. I understood this, and I could not blame him. Yet Hassan had another solution. If Abdullah collected the samples from Saraqeb, we would meet him in Bab al-Hawa, which was just across the border, inside Syria. This proposal was eagerly accepted

by all of us, at which point I began to explain the procedures Abdullah would have to follow.

'Make this very clear to him,' I told Hassan. 'He must
wear protective clothing when taking the samples; mask
and gloves are vital. He should take pictures and video
when he collects them and he should store the containers
in a sealed box, then place them in a cool box with lots of
ice, to keep the samples freezing cold. Without any of these
things, the samples might be useless.'

It was a big ask. Keeping the samples at a low temperature was going to be a struggle in this heat. But when
Hassan relayed all of this to Abdullah, it seemed that my
mad plan was going to go ahead. I felt exhilarated, as if
I was on a top-secret ops mission, which I suppose I was.
But there was no way I was going to tell anyone back home
what I was up to. I would be the last one to be having a
heart attack if they knew I was actually going to cross into
Syria.

With no time for second thoughts, I was soon jumping
into one of Hassan's convoy of trucks, and sat up front
with the man himself. In the back of the truck were the
goods that needed to be delivered. I just prayed that when
we returned it would also contain samples from Saraqeb.

We made our way to Reyhanli, the border crossing
point from Turkey into Syria, where there had recently been
a massive car bomb that had killed fifty-four people and
injured many more. *What are you doing, Hamish?* I sud-

denly asked myself. *You're crossing into a war zone with a man you've never met before.* But it was too late now.

Negotiating the border with surprising ease, we began the short journey to Bab al-Hawa. I had never before set foot in Syria so this gave me a chance to acclimatize myself. At this time the country was nowhere near as chaotic as it would later become. All of the roads still appeared to be in good working order, shops and restaurants were open, and children were playing in the streets. Unless you went looking for it, as I was, it was hard to tell that this was a country in the midst of a civil war. It was certainly a far cry from Iraq.

Despite things seeming remarkably calm I was now very much aware that if I got into trouble out here there would be no one I could call for help. This wasn't like Iraq or Afghanistan, where the West had boots and bases on the ground and you could call in a rescue team. There was no Western military presence here whatsoever. And even if there had been, I was now just a civvie. I had no support network. All I had was my mobile phone to call Julia, and I'm not sure how much help she could have been in such circumstances. Thankfully, the atmosphere didn't appear to be hostile and I had no intention of overstaying my welcome. This was going to be the definition of an in-and-out job. There would certainly be no sightseeing.

I was grateful that Hassan was good company. He almost delighted in having someone alongside him who had never before set foot in his country, to tell about its incredible heritage, particularly the ancient city of Palmyra, outside Homs, which boasted stunning temples and a Roman theatre. 'When this is all over, you must go,' he urged. Sadly, ISIS destroyed some of the site in 2015, decimating in the blink of an eye monuments and statutes that had stood for thousands of years.

Hassan was so engrossing that I was almost disappointed that the journey to Bab al-Hawa was so short. Just twenty minutes after crossing the border we had arrived. Things were now getting serious and I needed to have my wits about me. Although I wasn't even carrying a gun, so God knows what I was planning to do if things suddenly got out of hand.

We passed block after block of low-level, sand-coloured buildings, some of which had been levelled by bombs in the previous months. By and large the city still appeared to be operational, with traffic still on the roads and people still going about their daily business. It was a tribute to the endurance and the bravery of the Syrian people, all attributes they would sadly require in abundance in the years to come.

After checking a map, Hassan soon pulled up alongside an apartment block near a busy road. This was where we were due to meet Abdullah. Stepping out of the truck, welcoming the morning heat on my face, I was taking a look around when suddenly the man we were waiting for stepped out from a doorway. 'Abdullah!' Hassan happily exclaimed, as the two friends wrapped each other in a warm embrace. 'This is Hamish, the man I was telling you about.'

I smiled and shook his hand. It was clear we were both nervous. If the wrong parties were to find out what we were doing, then we would all be killed. There was no doubt about that. We also didn't know each other. All we each had to go on was Hassan's word, and I barely knew him. All the while I was on my guard, well aware that a Westerner was bound to attract attention. I knew that I did not have time to hang around. We needed to get the samples and get out of Dodge as soon as we could.

'Do you have the samples?' Hassan finally asked.

Abdullah nodded, handing a cool box over to me. 'What about the video and photographs?' I asked.

Taking out his phone, he showed me a video of him taking a sample from the bomb site. Kneeling over the hole, he took out chunks of earth and concrete, placing them into a plastic box, and then into the cool box I now had in my hands. As far as I could tell, the location was the same as I had seen in Ian Pannell's footage. It all looked entirely legitimate.

'I will send them to Hassan to give to you,' Abdullah promised.

It appeared we had what we came for. We thanked Abdullah for his help, and he wished us both well as we returned to the truck, to make our way back to the border. Opening the back door, looking for somewhere to hide the samples, I opened the cool box to get a better look. My heart sank. The ice keeping the samples cool had virtually all melted. There was no way to tell if the samples had been kept at the required temperature to make them an acceptable form of evidence. Looking at the state of them, I feared they might already be past the point of no return.

'We need ice!' I called out to Hassan, urgently explaining the situation. A little way down the road, he stopped outside a coffee shop and emerged soon after with a bag of ice to fill the box. I hoped this would keep the samples cool long enough for us to cross the border and get them to a contact at the OPCW, who could then verify whether they were still useful.

After hiding the samples in the back of the truck, we made our way back to the border, soon joining a queue of cars and trucks waiting to cross. All being well, we would be back at the hotel in less than fifteen minutes, having spent just under two hours in Syria.

However, as Abdullah had warned, the border checks leaving Syria were far more stringent than those we had faced on the way in. Guards were searching the backs of trucks and luggage, while also patting down all drivers and passengers. On the way in we had faced none of this. Suddenly my nerves got the better of me.

'I'm not sure this is a good idea,' I said.

'The security is always like this when leaving. It is not unusual,' Hassan replied.

That was little comfort to me. If I had been sure the samples were good enough, then it might have been worth the risk of taking them across, but I was already fearful that they were tarnished. As we moved closer to the guards, my mind suddenly flashed to a film I had seen in the cinema while at school, *Midnight Express*. In it, a young American student was arrested for smuggling drugs and sent to a Turkish prison. It was horrifying. My palms suddenly grew very sweaty and I found myself inadvertently grinding my teeth. *Think, Hamish! For Christ's sake, think!*

'We need to get rid of the samples,' I suddenly said.

'But we are almost there,' Hassan replied, as another car moved up in front of us.

'If we get caught with these samples, both of us will be facing a long time in jail.'

'I am aware of the risks,' Hassan said, fully intending to go ahead.

'I know you are, but I don't think the samples we have right now are worth it.'

This stopped him. 'They're no good?' he asked.

I shook my head. 'I don't think so.'

The car in front now took another nudge forward. Hassan sighed deeply, clearly frustrated. 'Then what do you want to do?'

'Dispose of them, and fast,' I said.

Shaking his head, Hassan finally accepted that this was our only choice. Jumping from the truck, I opened the back door, quickly retrieved the samples, ran to a grass verge, far away from any danger and out of view from the guards, and buried them in a small hole. Racing back to the truck, I hopped into my seat as Hassan moved us forwards once more, taking us towards the guards.

Moments later, they proceeded to search every inch of the truck, as well as us. It was clear they weren't messing around. I was certain that if we had kept the samples hidden in the back of the truck, there was a very good chance they would have been found.

Soon we were waved on our way through the border. I was relieved I had acted when I did, but I was still frustrated. The trip had been a total waste of time. I apologized to Hassan, who had so dearly wanted to get the samples out and nail Assad, but I think even he realized we had just had a lucky escape. As he dropped me back at the hotel, just before midday, we shook hands and promised to keep in touch. I was glad to have met him. But my troubles were not yet over.

Landing at Heathrow, I was not amused to hear the captain state over the tannoy, 'Ladies and gentlemen, sorry for the delay but British counter-terrorism police will soon be boarding to remove someone from the plane.' Tired and irritable, I thought to myself, *Which bloody idiot is this?* It turned out the bloody idiot they wanted was me.

Surrounded by police officers, I was frogmarched off the plane and then out through the terminal as if I was Osama bin Laden himself. Hauled into an interview room, I soon realized what this was all about.

'We believe you are carrying illegal substances from Syria, sir,' an officer declared.

'I have been to Syria but I'm certainly not carrying anything on me,' I truthfully replied, having not a clue how they might have obtained such information. I couldn't imagine that they knew about my brief foray into Syria, but I had of course been filmed speaking to the BBC about sarin from the border at Hatay. Perhaps that had been enough to put me on a watch list.

As they searched my case, apparently looking for traces of sarin, I noticed that they weren't wearing proper protective equipment. If I *had* been carrying anything, they could have become contaminated themselves. More worrying, it also seemed that they had no idea what they were looking for. Watching in disbelief, I could stand it no more. 'Do you know what sarin looks like?' I asked. It turned out they didn't have a clue. They didn't even realize it was a liquid. They thought it was a powder. Soon I was giving an impromptu lecture to the sheepish officers on what protective items they should be wearing to avoid contamination as well as what they should be looking for. I was shocked that the security in Britain's top airport, against something as dangerous as chemical weapons, was so poor. I was, however, released soon after without charge, which was certainly a relief after a challenging twenty-four hours.

Though my mission had failed, and the OPCW still could not get access into Syria, there was some progress. The UN was able to conduct an autopsy on the body of Mariam Khatib, the woman who had been treated in Turkey and had sadly died. Their subsequent report stated that the autopsy 'clearly indicated signatures of a previous sarin exposure'. The presence of sarin in biomedical samples was also confirmed by a French report in 2017. Nevertheless, nothing happened. No action whatsoever was taken against Assad.

My initial visit to Syria might not have gone to plan but I had learnt some valuable lessons, and I still felt I might be able to help. There was no getting away from the fact I felt re-energized, as if I had a purpose that must be fulfilled. I knew the situation in Syria and I knew the stakes. A humanitarian disaster was about to unfold unless something was done. Thankfully, I was soon contacted by somebody who thought I might be able to help as well. Heart condition or not, I had no hesitation in stepping forward, ready to plunge head first into a wild and crazy world that would soon dominate the front pages, as well as my life.

11

The Task Force

In the weeks that followed the attack in Saraqeb, Assad appeared to refrain from launching any further chemical attacks. But this certainly didn't mean things were improving – ISIS was now on the march in Syria and Iraq.

Shortly after the 2003 US-led invasion of Iraq, terrorist insurgencies had popped up all over the country. One of these was al-Qaeda in Iraq (AQI), formed by a Jordanian jihadist by the name of Abu Musab al-Zarqawi, aka the 'sheikh of the slaughterers'. With the blessing of Osama bin Laden, AQI soon became a major thorn in the coalition's side. However, after al-Zarqawi's death in 2006, at the hand of US forces, AQI had created an umbrella organization, Islamic State in Iraq (ISI). Yet without al-Zarqawi at the helm, ISI was steadily weakened by a surge in US troops as well as many Sunni Arabs rejecting the group for its brutality.

But in 2010 the group's fortunes changed, when Abu Bakr al-Baghdadi, a former US detainee, took charge, rebuilding ISI's capabilities. By 2013 the group had re-emerged as a significant presence and was once again carrying out dozens of attacks in Iraq. It had also joined the rebellion against President Bashar al-Assad in Syria, setting up the al-Nusra Front.

In April 2013, Baghdadi announced the merger of his forces in Iraq and Syria, with the official creation of the Islamic State in Iraq and Syria (ISIS). You won't be surprised to hear that the group's goal was to take over both countries, as well as other Muslim states, and form a caliphate, where its wicked brand of the Islamic religion would be enforced by brutal means.

Just weeks later, the Syrian city of Raqua, just a hundred miles from Aleppo, fell into ISIS's hands. Imposing their bastardized version of Sharia law, they executed any Alawites and Christians who refused to convert. Around a quarter of a million people fled scenes of pure horror, many ending up in refugee camps on the Turkish border. Meanwhile, ISIS began to move across northern Syria, pushing out the FSA and other opposition groups, showing their strength wherever they could, often in a bloodthirsty fashion.

While this was devastating for Syria and Iraq, it was also bad news for SecureBio. With ISIS on the march in Iraq, the Kurds were once more fighting for their independence. The region's probable descent into war meant that, for now at least, the Halabja contract would have to be postponed. This was a monumental blow to the business, and also very distressing for the families of the thousands of poor souls who remained buried in mass graves.

As we were trying to somehow plug this hole, I was approached by Dr Ghanem Tayara, a leading GP based in Birmingham. Dr Ghanem had spent a lot of time in Syria, helping to treat victims, and was now a director of the medical charity Union of Medical Care and Relief Organisations (UOSSM), which ran fifty hospitals in Syria. A coalition of humanitarian, non-governmental and medical organizations, UOSSM provided medical care to victims of war in Syria, regardless of their religion, ethnicity or political affiliation. It was extremely dangerous work – many UOSSM members had already been killed – and people such as Dr Ghanem did all of this for free, wanting nothing more than to help.

Knowing that I was a CBRN expert, and having seen me in the media, Dr Ghanem called me soon after the attack in Saraqeb with a proposition: 'Hamish, can you run some seminars in Syria to help our doctors understand how to identify and treat chemical injuries?' I thought this was a tremendous idea. Not many doctors in Syria were trained to deal with chemical injuries and, because of this, some had already died due to cross-contamination. Far more than the bombs and the bullets, it was the gas which really terrified them.

By now my family and business partners were aware that I had already paid a brief visit to Syria, something which had filled them with horror. It's fair to say that they were not overly enthused by this new idea, especially when the business had just suffered a major blow. But I made it clear that this trip was far from a jolly. The project had the potential to save lives and make a difference. Everyone understood that, but it was the rise of ISIS that made my business colleagues and family – and not least myself – extremely concerned. I promised to take extra precautions, never staying in Syria overnight, and to also wear a disguise. I'm not sure this totally convinced them but I at least went with their blessings.

When I arrived at the hotel in Hatay, in Turkey, it was clear that things in Syria had changed rapidly since my previous visit just a few weeks before. On my last visit, the hotel had been very quiet and the other guests had looked relatively normal. But now the hotel bar told a very different story. As I took the corner seat, where I had first met Hassan, I looked around and couldn't help but think it resembled the famous Mos Eisley Cantina from *Star Wars*, with its eclectic clientele, all drowning their sorrows and scheming in dark corners. While there were journalists from all corners of the globe, there were also arms dealers, spies, adventurers and I'm sure a smattering of people with links to terror organizations. I found it amusing to try to guess who was who, although they were all probably wondering what I was doing there as well.

The next morning, despite the worsened situation and the risk of kidnap, I popped my beta blockers and went outside for a run. Just because I was away there was no excuse not to keep fit, as well as to continue perfecting my Mo Farah running and breathing techniques. The scenery was beautiful, and I actually found it very peaceful. However, it was clear from some of the looks I got from journalists, as I passed them in the lobby in my running gear, that they thought I was insane. They didn't know the half of it.

Returning to my room, I put on a doctor's uniform and inspected my newly grown beard, completing my disguise. While it had been dangerous to be a Westerner in Syria before, now it was almost suicidal – reports had emerged of ISIS capturing and beheading any Westerners they could find. In November 2012, James Foley, a freelance American journalist had been kidnapped in the north of Syria on his way to Turkey. Not long after my visit, Alan Henning, a forty-seven-year-old taxi driver from Salford, was kidnapped at a checkpoint on his way to Aleppo, driving an aid-organization ambulance. A few months later, a video emerged of him being beheaded. And so, with my thick beard, I was now to be known as Dr Mohammed, a Muslim doctor, with a fake ID to back this up. I felt and looked ridiculous but there was no way I could risk wearing no disguise at all.

I walked downstairs and jumped into the UOSSM mini-bus waiting outside the hotel. Along with other doctors and medics, I crossed the border shortly after midday and set off for our destination: Aleppo.

The Syrian capital had been a magnet for trouble ever since the war had started. By the end of 2012 the rebels had seized much of the eastern and southwestern parts of the city, at which point the Syrian Army hit back, desperate to regain lost territory and wipe out the rebels. So began the so-called 'Battle of Aleppo'. While the situation waiting for us in Aleppo was sure to be grim, it was instantly clear that even the short journey there would not be an easy one.

Travelling on a stretch of highway known as the 'death road', I saw that Syria was now coming to resemble Iraq. To the side of the road, dumped in ditches, I saw burnt-out, bullet-ridden, overturned cars. In one I even saw the remains of its driver, the poor soul's decaying head resting against the steering wheel.

In some of the villages we passed I saw the reason for this carnage. From the roofs of some of the buildings, black ISIS flags, emblazoned with their distinctive white Arabic writing, were fluttering in the wind. Within a matter of weeks the terror group's tentacles had spread like a virus, infecting everywhere it touched. The villagers had no choice but to flee their homes and make for the border, or else face either converting to ISIS's uncompromising medieval religion or execution.

As I thought of the awful choice that had confronted these poor people, the bus suddenly came to a stop. Glancing out of the window I saw a chain strung across the road and several men, dressed head to toe in black. All were carrying automatic weapons. No one said a word. We all knew they were ISIS. It was my first chance to get a look at these bastards up close. They all looked so young. Most were no older than teenagers. No doubt many had been brainwashed, but I still despised them. I would have done anything to pop each of them in the head right then, but all I could do was sit tight and let our driver handle the situation, as he had advised. As we all sat in silence, he told the men we were all doctors. At this one of the guards took a stroll around the bus, looking at each of us through the windows. I kept my head down, hoping my new-grown beard would do the trick. It seemed to pass muster, as before my heart could really get racing we had been waved through. To say I was relieved was an understatement, which I think my colleagues found rather amusing.

'You know, ISIS are offering rewards for anyone who turns any Westerners over to them,' one man said.

'You are a strong British man, Hamish,' another chirped. 'We might get a good price for you!'

I joked back, 'As long as you split the reward with my wife, I don't think she will mind too much.' It was gallows humour but it gave us all a laugh and certainly broke the bubble of fear we had just been living in.

Soon after, we arrived in the capital, and I was shocked at what greeted me. Intensive bombing campaigns had turned large parts of the city to rubble, with heritage sites, mosques and areas of architectural wonder all unspared. Many of the roads were also impassable, adding more time on to our journey as our driver had to somehow navigate a new route, finding that one road after another no longer existed. As we navigated our way around the city, I saw that whole apartment blocks now lay abandoned, as did cars on the roads. People had just grabbed their belongings and fled. One block of buildings had its exterior walls blown out, revealing a child's pink bedroom. I prayed the inhabitants had managed to get out alive. All the while, the familiar smell of a war zone filled my nostrils: stale sewage. Sanitation in such places was all but impossible. In some places the smell was so strong I could almost taste it on my tongue.

Finally arriving at the hospital just after 3 p.m., I was led to a conference room where twenty to thirty doctors were already waiting for me. By this time there had already been two alleged chemical attacks in Aleppo, including the Khan al-Assal attack on 19 March 2013, which had killed and injured dozens of people. The doctors told me that they had been overwhelmed by this. They had never before had to treat those affected by a chemical attack and the hospital wasn't prepared for it. In the chaos, there had been no time to think about decontamination, they had just had to act or people would die. It was therefore unsurprising that some of the doctors became contaminated themselves.

After introducing myself, I quickly got down to work, appreciating that time was of the essence. At any moment these brave men and women, who worked all hours for little or no pay, could be called into action.

One of the key lessons I wanted to hammer home was the danger of cross-contamination, something the world is certainly far more aware of following the COVID-19 pandemic. It was vital that should they suspect they had come in contact with anything hazardous, they should avoid touching any surfaces or go near anyone else until they had washed themselves down with a chlorus solution. Even protective gloves were to be destroyed after use. They had to be thorough. If anyone did this half-heartedly, then the chemical could still contaminate them and others. But not everything was so straightforward.

In the event of a chemical attack, Porton Down had always recommended setting up a 'hot zone' for patients outside the hospital, which would help avoid further con-tamination. Yet as I suggested this, one of the doctors shot his hand in the air. 'You're saying this hot zone should be outside?' he said. I told him that was correct. 'But what about the snipers?' he replied. I hadn't thought of this.

The hospital was surrounded by fighting from all sides. If patients were placed outside, snipers in the buildings opposite would pick them off, as the doctors had already found to their cost. Such was the depravity of the snipers that it seemed they set themselves challenges, aiming for a certain body part each day. On one horrific occasion, they even shot a pregnant woman in the stomach, the bullet hitting the baby in the head. The X-ray of this act of evil was seen in newspapers all around the world.

If the snipers weren't enough of a threat, Syrian jets had also shown no qualms about dropping bombs on to hospitals. It was horrendous but a fact of life. The Porton Down model clearly wouldn't work in a place like this. All I could suggest was that the doctors house victims of chemical attacks in separate buildings. This would not eliminate the risk of cross-contamination but at least the victims would be safer than if they were out in the open.

At the end of my seminar, I gave my contact details to all of the doctors and told them to contact me should they have any questions, particularly in the event of a chemical attack. Wishing them all well, I was soon back in the minibus on my way back to the border. The country was now far too volatile for Westerners to stay the night. We had to be out by nightfall or we could be facing a very uneasy time indeed.

Leaving the darkening city behind, now only partially illuminated owing to power outages, we were soon out on the open road and looking forward to a stiff drink in the hotel bar, as well as a warm bath. I was well and truly exhausted. But it had been a very rewarding experience, and one I realized could prove to be invaluable in treating casualties in the weeks and months ahead.

Up ahead, in the darkness, I suddenly saw some headlights. Blocking the road was a truck, with two armed men, again dressed all in black, wielding their weapons. 'ISIS,' one of the passengers muttered. We all grimly nodded our heads, although we weren't too perturbed following our relatively easy passage earlier in the day. But this was to be anything but.

As our vehicle came to a stop, one of the men put the barrel of his gun to the driver's head and started shouting and screaming like a total lunatic. Our driver tried to remain calm but soon looked towards us. 'He wants everyone out,' he said. *You must be joking,* I thought. But there was nothing we could do, unless we wanted to be shot where we sat.

Slowly getting up and leaving the vehicle, I was conscious that I was the only Westerner in the group, even though I sported a decent beard and my ID said I was 'Dr Mohammed'. We were ordered to stand in a line, as one of the men shone a torch at each of us, apparently demanding our documents and wanting to know what we were doing. As he came closer, apprehension gripped my chest. *Don't have a heart attack now,* I thought. If my heart decided to play up, there was no way I was going to get out of this alive.

Two breaths in . . . Two breaths out . . . Two breaths in . . . Two breaths out . . .

I did this over and over, trying to remove myself from this stressful situation and somehow find some calm.

The ISIS thug continued to shine his torch into everyone's faces. I wondered if I could make a run for it, or better yet, take them both on. I didn't have a gun on me but even though these two were playing the part of terrifying terrorists I would have bet my last pound that they had never completed any sort of military training. Neither of them appeared that big either. I was sure I could definitely take one of them out, but what then?

Yet just as I was thinking this the light of the torch was suddenly in my face. With a wild glare, one of the thugs, who looked like a weasel, shouted at me. My mouth went dry. I didn't have a clue what he was saying but I had picked up a few of the words he had said to others in the line, at which they had said their names. Praying that this was what I was also being asked, I replied in Arabic, 'Dr Mohammed'. Again, the weasel shouted at me, this time from so close that I could smell his stale breath and catch the dead look behind his eyes. At this I pulled out my fake ID, again copying what others had done and hoping this was indeed what he wanted. Grabbing it from my hands, he looked down at it, then looked back at me. It seemed an age before the little weasel thrust the ID back into my hand and moved on to the doctor next to me. My disguise, and the fake ID, had just saved my life.

Hurriedly boarding the bus, after being forced to pay a 'toll', we were soon back on our way, happy to be getting out of this godforsaken place before nightfall. However, our troubles were not yet at an end.

As we neared the Turkish border, our driver shook his head in frustration, 'The border is closed.' We daren't go back but the longer we stayed on the Syrian side of the border, out in the open, the more likely it was that our luck would run out. Someone mentioned the idea of staying the night at the nearby refugee camp, which wasn't the most tantalizing prospect, but what other options did we have?

However, this suggestion did prompt a quite unbelievable turn of events. We learnt that in the camp there was a hole in the fence that could get us to the Turkish side of the border. Apparently, it was being used by the CIA to funnel aid and other items back and forth, and the Turks were, for now at least, turning a blind eye. I can't disclose how we learnt about this, but it seemed our best bet.

Entering the darkened refugee camp, we drove along a mud-covered road, past thousands of ragged, stained tents, whose dishevelled inhabitants loitered outside. This went on for as far as the eye could see. There were millions of them there, ordinary people, like you or me, all trying desperately to flee the war, and now they were trapped. It was horrendous. A true humanitarian disaster.

Suddenly turning off down a side track, we travelled for a few minutes in the pitch black before we reached the fence. The driver and one of the other men got out and pulled a section back. It seemed the legend was true. But I was still very aware of the overlooking watch towers, all manned by men toting machine guns. As we drove through the fence, and closed it behind us, a Turkish border patrol vehicle flashed its lights in front of us. With a machine gun at his side, the guard got out and barked at us in Turkish. Usually this would have been cause for alarm, but after our brush with ISIS I don't think any of us were too perturbed. Thankfully, after the driver explained the situation, and we all showed our passports, we were soon waved on our way.

It had been an intense day to say the least but it was not my last trip into Syria with UOSSM. In the months ahead I continued to train Syrian doctors, whether in Syria itself, at the Turkish border or even over Skype, ensuring they were fully prepared for any attack. And I was soon glad I had, as on 21 August 2013 Assad launched his most deadly chemical attack yet.

12

Crossing the Red Line

In the early hours of 21 August 2013, surface-to-surface rockets were fired at the Damascus suburb of Ghouta. One after another they kept coming, destroying buildings and blowing out doors and windows. Woken from their beds, those who were lucky enough to survive this initial onslaught ran to their basements to escape. As they did so, other rockets landed with a thud, but instead of exploding, these started to hiss before discharging an invisible gas. Catching on the light breeze, the gas wafted its way through all the blown-out doors, walls and windows, squeezing through any nooks and crannies, finally reaching the basements where many families were huddled together.

Unaware that the air was now poisoned with sarin, fathers, mothers, children and grandparents breathed it in. Seconds later they were gasping for air, their nerves shutting down one by one, forcing their bodies into spasm, then uncontrollable vomiting and then, finally, death.

Some escaped their basements but soon collapsed in the street, foaming at the mouth, their eyes rolling into the backs of their heads. Some tried to help them, frantically hosing them down with water, tearing off their clothes, in a desperate attempt to wash the sarin away. Others were told to put towels soaked with vinegar and lemon under their noses, hoping that this old wives' tale would somehow neutralize the evil agent.

Those who realized what was happening started screaming and crying, 'GAS! GAS! GAS!' Many now clambered to the top of their buildings, knowing that gas seeps down to the lowest point, hoping they could escape the invisible enemy. But even then they weren't safe, as mortar after mortar continued to rain down all around them. They were left with an impossible choice: stay upstairs and risk being bombed? Or go to the basement and risk being gassed? There was no right answer. Everywhere they turned they faced an appalling death.

Soon the hospitals were overwhelmed with casualties. Many of the doctors on call had attended my seminars, so thankfully they knew what they were dealing with, but such were the numbers of desperately ill people flooding through the doors it was all but impossible to follow procedures. What were they supposed to do when a mother frantically handed them a ten-month-old baby, frothing at the mouth? Their instant reaction was to take the child and try to wash it down, without a thought for themselves. It was hard to keep your head when all around you people were crying and screaming, desperately performing CPR on loved ones or looking around, lost.

Videos quickly uploaded to social media showed the world the horrifying aftermath in real time. Victims were once more shown to be suffering from symptoms attributable to sarin, while hundreds of body bags were lined up at morgues. One particular video that stuck in most minds was that of parents desperately trying to resuscitate their dead children, crying, sobbing, pleading for help. No words can truly convey the terror and desperation of being in a situation like this but perhaps if you just think hard enough, of someone you love dying the most appalling death, with no one able to save them, then perhaps you might get just a glimmer of what many families in Syria felt that day, and many more after.

It is thought that as many as 1,700 people died in that attack, but it was impossible to say how many would die or suffer from the after-effects in the weeks, months and years that followed. Seven out of nine doctors who had treated the survivors at our UOSSM clinic in East Ghouta died from secondary contamination. Some had not been aware that a chemical agent had been involved, as it was the first time they had encountered such an attack. Those who were aware selflessly continued to treat the patients anyway, irrespective of the danger to themselves. It was an unimaginable war crime, and it was later found that the sarin that had been used was even more potent than that used at Halabja.

Unsurprisingly, Russian President Vladimir Putin described claims that the Syrian government was responsible for the attack as 'utter nonsense'. He instead claimed that this was a 'false flag' attack by the rebels to provoke international military intervention. No one was buying this, no one with any sense anyway.

The White House revealed that their intelligence indicated 'with high confidence' that the Syrian government was responsible. Not only was there evidence of the Syrian regime preparing the weapons in the nearby Damascus suburb of Adra three days before but satellite images revealed these rockets being fired from the government-controlled territory towards Ghouta. The French and British governments also agreed with this assessment, with the French stating that 'the launch zone for the rockets was held by the regime while the strike zone was held by the rebels'. It was also widely known that while the rebels did not have access to chemical agents the Syrian military possessed more than 1,000 tonnes of the stuff, including several hundred tonnes of sarin.

Desperately scrambling to save face, Assad invited the OPCW to investigate the site, on the proviso that it was not allowed to determine who was responsible for the attacks. Meanwhile, governments in the West prepared to take military action, with the British Parliament set to vote on the matter on 29 August 2013.

For someone who had never had any interest in the politics of war, I now found myself at the heart of the political debate. With the vote fast approaching, I was determined to make myself available to any MPs who wanted an account from someone who had actually investigated previous attacks in Syria and was a CBRN expert.

The week that followed saw me up at all hours, whether speaking to MPs on the telephone, visiting them at their constituency offices or even meeting with them in Parliament itself. Those who were particularly interested to know more included Andrew Mitchell, renowned for being vocal on humanitarian matters, as well as John Woodcock and Alison McGovern.

Since the attack on Saraqeb, when no action had been forthcoming from the West, I explained to MPs, things had escalated in Syria at a terrifying pace. There had since been reports of four more chemical attacks, with the attack at Ghouta the most horrifying of all. I felt it was clear that if we once more allowed this to go unchallenged then things would only get worse, in Syria, and possibly beyond.

However, after outlining this to any MPs who were willing to listen, and showing them the photographs and video footage from Ghouta, most returned with the standard response: 'We don't want another Iraq on our hands, Hamish.'

I had a degree of sympathy for their dilemma. In hindsight, the invasion of Iraq had proven to be a disaster. No weapons of mass destruction were ever found, at least not at the levels the government had indicated Saddam had at his disposal. It had also opened up the gates of hell in the Middle East. Terrorist groups such as Al Qaeda and ISIS had surged as Iraq was torn apart by foreign occupation, costing billions of pounds and millions of lives in the process, including those of British soldiers. I don't think there was anyone in Britain who wanted to repeat those mistakes.

Yet I felt the situation in Syria was very different. While there had been plenty of talk of WMDs in Iraq, none were ever found or deployed. In Syria, we had already seen that chemical weapons had been used on at least twenty-four occasions since the war had started. There were already estimated to be around 2,000 deaths attributable to chemical attacks, with thousands more injured. It was also impossible to say how many more would continue to suffer in the years to come.

Obama's 'red line' warning against the use of chemical weapons had clearly been crossed. I explained to MPs that this 'red line' had actually existed since the end of the First World War, and that anybody who had used chemical weapons should expect to face severe repercussions, whether they were a signatory to an anti-chemical weapon convention or not. If we did not act, we were effectively giving the green light not only to Putin and Assad but to every despot and terrorist around the world: chemical and biological weapons would now be fair game.

While some MPs were reluctant to take firm action, it seemed that most of the British public also had little appetite to get involved. An *Observer* opinion poll conducted just before the vote showed how strongly the public were against military intervention. Some 59% of voters said the UK's recent entanglements in Iraq and Afghanistan had made them more reluctant to support military interventions by UK forces abroad. This was particularly true among those over 55, 70% of whom said they had been put off by the way these actions had turned out. As such, 60% of voters said they were opposed to the UK taking action in Syria, with the most popular option being to put greater diplomatic pressure on the Syrian regime, such as economic sanctions. Such feelings clearly played on the minds of the MPs who were set to vote.

I understood that to many this was just yet another war, in the far-off Middle East, that people wanted to keep at arm's length. I understood their reluctance to get involved. Indeed, if I had not been to Syria myself and actually seen what was going on, maybe I would have been of the same mind. Yet I believed that there was a real danger that elements of this could soon be on our doorsteps. Syria is a lot closer to us than most people think. It is a Mediterranean rather than Middle-Eastern country, bordering

Turkey. Millions of Syrians were already displaced, hungry, wounded and without shelter. Thousands of refugees were already trying to cross the border into Turkey and from there into Europe. It was clear that before long this would become an influx and Europe would struggle to cope. Worse yet, I was certain that many terrorists would be hiding amongst this influx, using the opportunity to carry out attacks on European cities. If we acted now, we could help the Syrian people, while also preventing the fallout from reaching our shores. There was also a real chance to quickly put an end to this ever-escalating conflict. In my opinion, Assad's use of chemical weapons had been a last throw of the dice to try to stay in control. The rebels had been gaining ground in Ghouta and were now only a few miles from his inner sanctum. Many believed the regime was about to fall. If we struck now, the war could all be over.

While I did my best to outline the situation to any MPs willing to listen, I also found myself in demand by the media. I was happy to speak to whomever I could so that the public, and any watching MPs, would have as much information as possible. But I soon found myself up against a wall of Russian propaganda. For the first time I saw how the likes of Twitter was being used to spread disinformation, which conspiracy theorists and what I like to call 'useful idiots' were all too keen to gobble up. By the term 'useful idiots', I refer to a bunch of wayward professors, who are employed by some of the best universities in the UK. From the comfort of their wood-panelled offices in some of our great cities, they spout rubbish about chemical attacks in support of Russia and the Syrian regime and against the UK, France and the US in particular. I find it abhorrent that my taxes are used to pay these deniers of such despicable crimes against humanity and I try to challenge them on their dangerous theories at every opportunity.

Much of the propaganda revolved around Russia's claim that it was terrorist organizations that had actually been responsible for the attack in Ghouta. They'd also claimed that this was a false flag operation to encourage the West to attack Assad. This was, of course, total nonsense. Remnants of the rockets that had been used in the attack had been recovered, and arms experts had identified some as Soviet-era 140mm surface-to-surface artillery rockets, known as the M-14, which the Syrian military was known to have in its possession and which could carry 2.2kg of sarin. Others were identified as 330mm rockets, compatible with the 333mm Falaq-2 launcher produced by Iran, which the Syrian government was also known to possess. Video footage also emerged appearing to show Syrian troops using Falaq-2 systems to launch similarly adapted rockets in previous attacks.

It was disheartening to see so many conspiracy theorists on social media be drawn to such outlandish stories and then eagerly share them with followers who didn't know any better. However, I was stunned at how the mainstream media were also taken in by this. Perhaps the most shocking case was the *New York Times* allowing Vladimir Putin to write an op-ed, speaking directly to the American people. I thought this was grossly irresponsible. I could understand them publishing an interview with Putin, in which they could have challenged his claims, but allowing him to write a column, totally unchallenged, only gave his wild conspiracies legitimacy in some eyes. In just a few years the same newspaper would, of course, become vehemently anti-Putin, alleging that he had meddled in the 2016 US election. I found this all a bit rich after it had allowed the man free rein to spread his lies about Syria.

Perhaps just as disconcerting as so many people appearing to fall for Russian propaganda was the fact that so many MPs also appeared to be playing politics with the issue. It seemed that the leader of the opposition, Ed Miliband, was particularly determined to take the opposing position to the government, come what may. It was clear that there had been multiple uses of chemical weapons by Assad during the war; it was also clear from all of the evidence emerging that he was responsible for the incident in Ghouta. Yet this wasn't enough for Miliband. He demanded further evidence and declared there would have to be a 'very significant change' in circumstances to allow Britain to join any operation in Syria. I wasn't quite sure what he was waiting for. All the evidence was there. We knew Syria had significant chemical capabilities, while intelligence, video footage, photographs, witness testimony and experts all made very clear that sarin had been used on numerous occasions. Unlike Iraq, Syria did actually have WMDs and was using them on a regular basis.

Miliband also said that Labour would only support military action against the Assad regime if Britain's national security was threatened or terror organizations gained possession of large stockpiles of chemical weapons. I found this particularly baffling. We had an opportunity to stop these events from ever taking place. Why would you take such a risk and not act? By sitting back at this juncture, we could be inviting a similar attack upon ourselves somewhere down the line. To my mind, he appeared to be paralysed by fear of repeating the mistakes of Iraq.

Most naïvely of all, Miliband advocated that military action should only be taken following a vote by the UN Security Council. On the face of it, this seemed perfectly sensible. After all, it seemed that invading Iraq without a UN resolution had been a particularly foolhardy thing to do. But getting a UN vote passed in these circumstances was nigh on impossible.

The UN Security Council has five permanent members: Russia, the United Kingdom, the United States, France and China – as well as 10 non-permanent members. For the Security Council to pass a vote, there must be nine votes in favour and none of the five permanent members must vote against. Therefore, even if there are nine votes in favour, one of the five can use its vote against to block the vote from passing. This was a privilege Russia had already used in relation to Syria, and would continue to use repeatedly, to stop military action, investigations, sanctions and even aid. By February 2020 it had voted fourteen times against any sort of action in Syria. It was for this reason that other European countries, as well as the US, were now looking to take action without going to the UN. Miliband must surely have been aware of this.

Despite all of this, Miliband instructed his MPs to vote against the government motion for military action. Watching the debate on television, I could see that the government was fighting an uphill battle. David Cameron's opening speech certainly didn't help matters. He rambled and didn't ever seem to get to the root of the matter: that if we didn't act now, then these horrendous weapons would not only continue to be used on the civilian population in Syria but could also soon reach our shores. He also didn't make clear that though Assad and Putin might very well have been targeting terrorists, they were killing thousands of innocent civilians in the process, often with outlawed weapons. In any event, how could we hold the moral high ground if we allowed such weapons to be used on our enemies?

But as speech after speech raised the spectre of another Iraq, and demanded more evidence, it became clear that the government was going to lose the vote, which they did, by an opposition majority of thirteen, with dozens of Tory MPs joining forces with Labour. By doing so, David Cameron became the first prime minister to lose a vote proposing military action since Lord North in 1782.

Without the support of a key ally, President Obama now faltered. Having been advocating military action, and looking set to gain Congressional support, he now changed tack. On 10 September 2013 he announced that the Syrian government had accepted a US–Russian negotiated deal to turn over 'every single bit' of its chemical weapons stockpile for destruction. It had also declared its intention to finally join the Chemical Weapons Convention, so such destruction could be overseen and investigated by the OPCW, which would also have the authority to inspect any sites in Syria, should there be reports of any further chemical attacks. It was a rare instance of a deal that both Russia and the US could realistically sell as a successful outcome, while the UN Security Council also backed it, on the proviso that it would impose measures under Chapter 7 of the UN Charter, which deals with sanctions and authorization of military force, in the event of noncompliance.

At this everyone patted themselves on the back and considered the matter as good as closed. When the OPCW's report into Ghouta finally came out, it confirmed sarin had been used, and while it was not authorized to identify the perpetrators, it certainly provided enough information to make it very clear who was responsible. By examining the debris field and the impact area where the rockets had struck, the inspectors were able to calculate their trajectories 'with a sufficient degree of accuracy'. When subsequently plotted on a map, Human Rights Watch said, the missile trajectories began at a large military base on Mount Qassioun, known to be home to the Syrian Republican Guard 104th Brigade.

The OPCW was awarded the 2013 Nobel Peace Prize for its involvement in Syria, and in the summer of 2014 it confirmed that Syria's 'declared' chemical stockpile had been removed from the country. The OPCW had also overseen the destruction of thirteen mobile and stationary chemical weapon production, mixing and filling facilities. Assad's chemical capabilities had apparently been destroyed, just as he had promised. While the civil war rumbled on, chemical attacks would at least be consigned to the past.

But a few months later I received a phone call from an old friend:

'Hamish, there has been another chemical attack. Can you help us?'

13

Getting a Sample

In the weeks that had followed the April 2013 attack on Saraqeb, when I had been asked by Dr Ghanem to help train Syrian doctors, the events of my trip to Bab al-Hawa with Hassan were still very much on my mind.

I had found to my cost that gathering samples from Syria was a particularly daunting challenge, and at this point the OPCW was also still unable to enter the country to investigate. While I was determined to try again, I realized that not only would it remain difficult to get the samples across the border but it was also becoming too dangerous for me to venture very far into Syria.

Getting to Aleppo was soon out of the question; the Bab al-Hawa Hospital in Idlib Province was now the furthest I could travel. Just twenty minutes from the border town of Reyhanli, Idlib was one of the few remaining strongholds keeping ISIS and Assad at bay. Beyond there, I was aware that it would be all but impossible for me to try to reach the site of a chemical attack.

However, I realized that I could help train the doctors, who were often first on the scene of any such attack, to take the samples themselves. This would also ensure that they were fresh, with little chance of decay or decontamination, which had caused me to throw away the Saraqeb samples.

Alongside Dr Alastair Hay, a world-renowned toxicologist from Leeds University, I ran a series of seminars to teach the doctors about the legal aspects of collecting samples, so that they would stand up under the strictest scrutiny. Together we demonstrated how blood, tissue, teeth, bones, clothes and soil samples were to be placed in special plastic bags and then put in triple-sealed containers to avoid contamination. Pictures of the samples were then to be taken on a digital camera to record the time, date and GPS location where they had come from. This was to prove that the samples were actually taken from the location where the bomb had been dropped. For the evidence to be admissible it was vital that the doctors followed these directions to the letter. Every detail was critical. If any link in the chain of evidence should break, it would make a sample worthless. I knew that people would be risking their lives in order to get these samples, so it was very important that they understood exactly what was required.

However, as I knew first-hand, getting samples to the border and smuggling them across was extremely problematic. As I had told Hassan's friend, the samples had to be kept below 17 degrees at all times. They couldn't just be hidden in, say, a doctor's pocket. They had to be kept in a cool box, which was obviously a hefty piece of kit and hard to hide. However, by now the roads were often blocked by Syrian soldiers, determined to stop the outside world from knowing what was going on, not to mention the thugs of AQ and ISIS. Anyone found with such an item could expect to arouse suspicion, and, if inspected, faced the prospect of being shot dead on the spot.

Even if, after all this, good-quality samples were to get across the border, there was no guarantee the world would act. This was emphatically seen in 2019 when Assad used chemical weapons against rebel-held areas that were controlled by ISIS. Doctors treating patients were able to get samples out, following which they proved positive for chlorine, but the West still turned a blind eye, claiming there were gaps in the chain of evidence to avoid taking action. I found this excuse to be a little too convenient, but I knew full well the reasoning behind it. It would be seen as political suicide if they were to punish Assad for killing members of ISIS, even if chemical weapons had been used.

Facing such obstacles, many of the doctors were wary about risking their lives if no one was going to act. At this I explained that, during the Bosnian and Kosovo wars, many Bosnians had felt deserted by the West, as the civilians in Syria did and still do. But sixteen years after the war had ended, the generals who had committed war crimes were now in prison, having been convicted by the International Criminal Court (ICC) in the Hague. The evidence that the doctors collected now could, in time, put Assad and his henchmen behind bars too. We might not see any immediate results, but in time they would come. I was sure of that.

It was during one of these seminars that I met an extraordinary young man by the name of Houssam Alnahhas. His story was remarkable. He told me that he had always wanted to be a doctor. From a young age, helping others was his passion. As such, he and his family were overjoyed when in 2006 he was accepted to study medicine at Aleppo University. However, in 2012, and just a few months before his graduation, the war had erupted in the city.

Houssam decided to abandon his studies for the foreseeable future and help. Along with some of his friends and professors, he created the Light of Life medical team to treat casualties. However, being a doctor and treating rebels was dangerous. Assad had made it quite clear that anyone helping rebels in any way would also be considered the enemy. It was for this reason that many hospitals were bombed in Syria. Because of this, Houssam and his colleagues had to operate in the shadows, changing their names and using unregistered phone numbers. Yet in just a few months they helped to save hundreds of lives, all the while avoiding detection.

But in June 2012, disaster struck when three of the team were arrested and executed by the Syrian government.

Houssam was distraught yet furious. He learnt that they had been tortured, their nails extracted and their limbs broken, before they were shot in the head and their bodies burnt. The day after Houssam received this news, he angrily emerged from the shadows and addressed a major demonstration. Wearing his uniform, he told the crowd that three young doctors had lost their lives, all because Assad did not want them to treat anyone who opposed him. To the cheers of the crowd, Houssam told them that despite this he and the other doctors involved with the Light of Life would do all they could to help the rebels.

Shortly afterwards, as Houssam and a friend were shopping for groceries, they were stopped by three armed men. Placed in handcuffs at gunpoint they were taken to a detention centre, where Houssam and his friend were stripped naked, bound and forced to lie facedown in a dungeon. Then the beating started. Every inch of Houssam's body was beaten black and blue as the men repeatedly asked, 'Who are the other doctors you are working with?' Refusing to answer, Houssam was soon almost unconscious from the beating, upon which his limp body was dragged to a small, dark cell containing fifty-three other people, who were also wounded or dying.

When Houssam came around, despite the fact he had been badly beaten himself, he tried his best to treat anyone who was suffering. However, without medicine or equipment it was often a lost cause. A thirteen-year-old boy who had been repeatedly beaten about the head in a torture chamber was continually vomiting. When Houssam told the guards the boy probably had a bleed on the brain and needed medical attention, he was told, 'Go to hell.' The next day the boy died.

Houssam and his friend were convinced that they would never get out of this place. They waited for the day when, like their three friends, they would be shot in the head. Yet after seventeen days spent in the cell and being beaten in the dungeon, Houssam was shocked to hear one of the guards call his name. To his surprise, he was told that he and his friend were being released. It turned out that his family had managed to pay a bribe.

Upon his release, Houssam immediately travelled to Damascus to be with his mother and father but the sense of injustice would not leave him. All the while the situation throughout the country was getting worse. When he had recovered from his ordeal, Houssam decided that he must return to Aleppo to help. But he knew his parents would not let him leave. To go to Aleppo now was suicide, especially if you were already a marked man.

Houssam decided to leave his family home in the middle of the night, so that his parents would not be able to stop him. Creeping to the door, he found it was locked and the keys were gone. When he turned around, he found his mother holding them. Pulling out a knife, she placed it in Houssam's hand and raised it to her chest. 'Kill me,' she begged. 'I cannot live waiting for someone to call me to tell me you are dead.' Houssam replied, 'You raised me to do this and you know it's right.' 'But what about me?' she cried. 'Please think about me.' Looking into her eyes, Houssam pulled the knife away. 'Mum, I love you,' he said. 'But you know my decision and you know you can't stop me.' With that, he calmly took the keys from his mother's shaking hand, opened the door and left for Aleppo.

Working as a first-response medic, Houssam often treated the victims of air strikes and barrel bombs that had been loaded with TNT explosive. Then a nerve agent attack on the city's Khan al-Assal district in March 2013 switched him on to the threat of chemical weapons. Most medics were unprepared to treat such injuries and it was certainly not something he had learnt in university. Such was the Assad regime's determination to stamp out the spread of information that some doctors were not even aware that chemical weapons had been used.

Houssam was determined to change this, particularly after it became clear that the West would not be riding to the rescue any time soon. Pulling together other interested medics, he established the initial CBRN Task Force to put in place procedures to react to a chemical attack. Having heard of my work with doctors, he got in touch with me via Skype and soon after we met for the first time at a seminar in Bab al-Hawa Hospital.

I liked Houssam from the get-go. He was very articulate

and spoke near perfect English, but in particular I liked his energy and positivity. He was one of those people who would go above and beyond to reach a goal. No matter the question and no matter the circumstances, the answer was always: 'Yes!' I've always found that the best sort of person to deal with is the one who looks for the positive rather than the negative. I will forgive almost any shortcoming if somebody has a positive attitude. I have no truck with the negatively minded.

Houssam asked if I could get involved with his CBRN Task Force, which matched my own ideas for how to treat victims and collect samples. I was only too delighted to help in any way that I could. Houssam and his doctors said they wanted to collect samples from chemical attacks but did not know what to do with them. At this stage they didn't entirely trust the UN, or the OPCW, to test them. With Russia continually using its veto and the West refusing to act, they felt that any samples they did collect would disappear. They therefore wanted to give them to someone they thought they could trust. That person turned out to be me.

So we worked out a procedure. Should there be a chemical attack, Houssam or someone from the Task Force would try to get to the site as quickly as possible. They would collect the samples, then high-tail it to the border, where I would be waiting at the other side to test them. In principle, it all sounded good. They knew that they would only have to be successful just the once and then the whole world would finally know that Assad was a war criminal. That was all they wanted. And in Houssam's words, 'It's an honour to risk our lives for such a cause.'

However, after the August 2013 Ghouta attack and Syria finally signing the Chemical Weapons Convention, there were no further incidents in the months that followed. Even I began to think that maybe it had dawned on Assad that any further use of chemical weapons would see him face the mother of all consequences. He had barely escaped by the skin of his teeth after Ghouta. If there was a next time, there would be hell to pay, especially as Syria was now a CWC signatory.

As things seemed to have settled down in this respect, and after a hectic few years here, there and everywhere, I thought it was about time my family and I enjoyed a holiday together. In April 2014 we finally found the time to do so, setting off for a skiing trip in France. It was wonderful. For the first time in years I felt myself totally relax and I loved bombing around the slopes with the kids, taking in the fresh air and the awe-inspiring scenery. I aimed to totally switch off my brain for a few days and forget all of the stresses of the world, not even bothering to read the news.

But then I received the message from Houssam: 'Hamish, there has been another chemical attack. Can you help us?'

'Where?' I asked, stunned that this should be happening again, particularly as Assad had declared his chemical stockpile to the UN and the OPCW was well on the way to destroying it all.

'Kafr Zita and Talmenes,' he replied. I knew these were rebel-held areas near Damascus. But if Assad had given up all of his chemical stockpile to the OPCW, how had such an attack been possible?

Houssam told me that on 11 April 2014 a bomb had been dropped on Kafr Zita at around 6 p.m. Plummeting to the ground, it had exploded its noxious payload on impact, and a toxic yellow vapour subsequently billowed through the town, seeping into homes and leaving families choking and gasping for breath. Though doctors battled to treat the effects of the gas, which had burnt the lungs of the people who ran, crawled or were carried through the doors of the field clinic, more than 150 died in total. The town was hit again on the 12th and the 16th, while two days later a gas-filled barrel was lobbed from a helicopter at night and landed so close to the local hospital that the doctors and nurses themselves became casualties.

Three days later, only thirty miles away in the village of Talmenes, another attack wounded hundreds, while three generations of one family were killed when a gas-filled barrel bomb was dropped on their home in Sarmin. Sheltering in their basement, they might have been safe from a conventional bomb, but the density of the gas caused it to seep to the lowest point in the building, smothering them all to death.

Immediately after the attack in Talmenes, Houssam had heard from the doctors on the scene that casualties were displaying unusual symptoms: eye and skin irritation, respiratory distress, a bloody froth from the mouth. These weren't symptoms they recognized as sarin but instead seemed to indicate exposure to chlorine.

Suddenly, it all made sense. While Assad might very well have given up his declared stockpile, including all his nerve agents, he had instead purchased 20,000 containers of chlorine from China, under the pretence that it was to be used to clean the country's water supply, as well as in the plastic, pulp, paper, pesticide and pharmaceutical industries. Using chlorine for these purposes was not illegal, and even for a country that was in the middle of a civil war it seemed a perfect reasonable purchase. However, Assad was now using chlorine-filled barrel bombs in acts of war, which was certainly against the Chemical Weapons Convention that he had only just signed.

'I think I can get to Talmenes and take samples,' Houssam continued. 'Will you be able to meet me in Gaziantep to collect them?'

I looked at my family, who were all preparing themselves for another day on the slopes. I knew how disappointed they would be if I left now, but what choice did I have? Houssam was going to risk his life to get these samples to me, which might very well prove that Assad had thrown the mercy of the world in its face. This might be our only chance. I had to go. Thankfully, while my family was disappointed that I was cutting my holiday short, they recognized just how important this could be, and they were also relieved that I wouldn't have to set foot in Syria myself.

Less than forty-eight hours later, and just a few days after the Talmenes attack, I waited nervously on the Turkish side of the Syrian border near Gaziantep, an industrial town that had recently been swelled by the arrival of over one million refugees. With me was Ruth Sherlock, a *Daily Telegraph* journalist who wanted to cover the story and ensure everything was above board. I thought it was vital that this was all documented properly, and I was only too happy to have the support and company of Ruth, who is a fiercely intelligent and thorough journalist.

By now the border was more intimidating than ever. Before us was a deep ditch, and then mile upon mile of 20-metre-high fences, dotted with watch towers every 500 metres, all manned by automatic machine guns. Behind the fence was no-man's land, covered in land mines. It was a fearsome sight, clearly designed to prevent any more refugees flooding across the border – 200,000 having recently crossed in a twenty-four-hour period. It was also designed to ensure any undesirable elements were confined to Syria, as the country was beset by foreign jihadis. I just had to hope that Houssam had a plan to get the samples across the border, but even before that he faced a number of challenges. Hours earlier we had heard unconfirmed reports that other doctors from the Task Force who had recently visited the town in an attempt to collect samples had been killed for doing so. The Syrian regime was now well aware of what people were doing and showed no mercy should they catch anyone in the act.

Before setting off on his mission, I again reminded Houssam of all the procedures he had to follow: triple-bagging, photographs, video footage and GPS locations, with metadata to show the time the samples were collected – and, of course, the samples had to be kept below 17 degrees in a cool box. It was vital that he strictly followed these procedures so that the samples would be admissible as evidence. I also told him that the key was getting samples from the barrel bomb itself. As most of it would have evaporated by now this was the most likely area to still have the highest concentration of chlorine.

'Wish me luck,' he said, before setting off.

'I'll pray for you,' I replied.

From Bab al-Hawa Hospital, Houssam, with two of his colleagues, a physician and a pharmacist, began the two-hour drive to Talmenes. Getting to the town would not be easy. They would have to cross a government-controlled area, all the while carrying the sample-collecting kit and the cool box. Time was also of the essence. The chlorine attack on Talmenes had occurred just a few days earlier. Houssam was desperate to reach the site as quickly as possible in order to collect a good-quality sample.

Thankfully, the trip to Talmenes was relatively uneventful. They passed through government checkpoints with no issue at all and were soon at the site of the attack, which Houssam told me smelt like a swimming pool. Chlorine was clearly still present, albeit not at levels dangerous to breathe in, but this at least boded well for the sample collection.

Identifying the remains of the barrel bombs, Houssam saw that one of them had inscribed on it 'Cl2', the chemical symbol for chlorine gas. He took some pictures of this, while he also took soil samples and, as we had discussed, triple-bagged them before placing them in a cool box in his car. He also took GPS readings from where the samples had been taken, as well as filming those readings, the surrounding area and the site itself. Absolutely nothing was left to chance. It was all textbook stuff.

Houssam and his colleagues then travelled to the hospital in Saraqeb, where patients were recovering from the attacks. On inspecting the desperately ill patients in the ICU ward, they found that all of their injuries were the same. There were no external wounds, just respiratory distress and irritation of the eyes and skin. Collecting blood, stool and urine samples, they also recorded interviews with some of the casualties, taking copies of the results of their lab tests as well as the X-rays of their lungs.

Once they had finished, Houssam called me. 'I have what we need,' he declared. 'I am on my way to the border.' This was great news. All being well he would be with us within two hours.

However, two hours later there was still no sign of him. When I called, it went straight to voicemail. 'Houssam,' I said, leaving a message, 'call me when you get this. Let me know you're all right.' But there was nothing. I nervously watched every vehicle that came through the crossing in hope. As yet another hour passed without news, I was beginning to fear the worst. Soon the border would be closing and I didn't fancy Houssam's chances if he had to keep the samples safe overnight, if he was even still alive.

As the minutes ticked by, and with the border set to close, I saw some headlights approaching. Praying this was Houssam, I peered into the car, relieved to see it was my friend and his two colleagues! Exhausted, dishevelled and with their nerves shot, they had made it. 'Do you have the samples?' I asked, to which Houssam nodded, but he had endured a hell of an ordeal to get them to me.

Just as they had set off from the hospital, they had heard the sound of a helicopter above them. They knew that the Syrian regime were the only forces who had access to air power and the helicopter seemed to be following them. Word had clearly got out that Houssam and his colleagues had been collecting samples, and they were now targets. This was no doubt the fate that had befallen the other doctors who had reportedly lost their lives trying to get samples out.

Roaring down the road, they tried to shake off the helicopter but it continued to give chase. Knowing that it was only a matter of time before it opened fire or dropped a bomb on them, Houssam turned off the headlights and suddenly pulled the car into a ditch off the road, hiding behind the wreckage of other cars. In the darkness they waited, huddled into their seats, the only sound that of the helicopter whirring around and around above, apparently trying to find them. If it had chosen to drop a bomb, there would have been no escape, but mercifully it gave up after twenty minutes.

Finally, when all was quiet, they left the ditch and, with their headlights still off, made their way to the border as quickly as possible, this time avoiding any trouble. But at the border there was another challenge: getting the samples across. I knew from bitter experience that the Turks were not particularly receptive to this, but Houssam and his friends were prepared.

Knowing this would be an issue, Houssam had previously made several trial runs across the border and back. Cool boxes were always bound to catch attention but when disguised as a suitcase, full of clothes, with samples kept in hidden compartments, more often than not it got through. This was the plan, and it looked set to work until they saw that an X-ray machine was now in place, to scan all luggage. Not only would this spot the hidden compartments but the X-ray could also damage the samples, making them inadmissible.

As Houssam had come this far, he decided there was no turning back now. While his colleagues placed cases on to the X-ray belt, Houssam confidently walked past, his jacket covering the cool box he pulled alongside him. It was hardly James Bond stuff but, unbelievably, it worked. No doubt at this late hour the guards were more interested in going home for the night. Perhaps the helicopter delaying Houssam's arrival had proved to be a benefit after all.

As Houssam handed over the samples, I checked their condition. They appeared to be very well preserved, and all the steps that had been taken were in line with those required by the OPCW. I was thrilled. Yet the proof would now be in the pudding. We now had to see if they contained any trace of chlorine, as we all suspected.

There was no way I could just board a plane and take the samples back to Britain, so I analysed them at the only place I knew to be safe: the flat roof of our hotel. With Houssam and Ruth watching, I ensured we all stayed upwind, as the samples were still likely to be toxic. Wearing my protective suit, and keeping a protective respiratory hood nearby, in case the wind changed and blew gases from the samples into my face, I set up the test and divided the samples into two. I would test one set myself, while we had arranged for the other set to be collected by a contact we trusted from the OPCW, so that they could also verify the results.

I opened the pot of earth from Talmenes, put it in a sealed plastic bag – called the 'headspace' – and then placed it in a mini WARN tester, a sophisticated machine that can detect even one particle per million of chlorine and ammonia in the air. The machine gave a few short perfunctory beeps. We watched with bated breath, then the tempo of the beeps increased.

'What does it mean?' Houssam asked as I looked at the results.

'It means it's found traces of chlorine and ammonia,' I replied. Even days after the attack, when most of the chlorine would have evaporated, it was clear that it had originally been delivered in a very high dose.

Just to reaffirm the results, I also subjected the samples to a separate litmus test. When chlorine gas comes in contact with water, it produces hydrochloric acid. When I mixed a small part of each sample with water, each test showed abnormally high acidity levels.

There was now no doubt whatsoever. Once more the Syrian population had been subjected to a chemical attack, despite all promises and denials to the contrary.

'Well done,' I smiled at Houssam. 'You did it!'

At this he nodded, showing little sign of emotion. While he was, of course, elated that his efforts had not been in vain, and that this bombshell evidence would prove Assad and Putin to be liars, he was also deeply saddened. It was clear that his countrymen had been subjected to another appalling attack, and would continue to suffer, unless something was now done. But this was unequivocal evidence. There could be no turning back now.

The *Daily Telegraph* revealed the results of the test on its front page and called for an urgent investigation. At this then-Prime Minister David Cameron called for the OPCW to investigate these attacks as a matter of utmost urgency. However, when OPCW inspectors tried to get to Kafr Zita, they had to turn back after coming under armed attack. With conditions clearly too dangerous to investigate, the OPCW decided that it would collate all available evidence in a so called 'fact-finding mission' before releasing a report. This evidence included everything that Houssam had collected and handed over.

The OPCW released preliminary reports in June and September 2014, which 'concluded, with a high degree of confidence, that chlorine had been used as a weapon in Syria'. But once again it could not name those it felt were the perpetrators.

However, on 7 August 2015, with the UN and the OPCW recognizing the need to identify who was responsible for such attacks, the Joint Investigative Mechanism

(JIM) was established by the UN Security Council through Resolution 2235. This aimed to 'identify to the greatest extent feasible, individuals, entities, groups or governments who were perpetrators, organizers, sponsors or otherwise involved in the use of chemicals as weapons, including chlorine or any other toxic chemical, in the Syrian Arab Republic'. While this would be a 'non-judicial mechanism', it would at the very least show the world at long last who the UN and the OPCW felt was responsible.

In August 2016, the OPCW released its final fact-finding report on the matter, using the JIM procedure for the first time. It said that it had 'compelling confirmation' that a toxic chemical had been used 'repeatedly' as a weapon in Syria, while for the first time it also pointed the finger at the Syrian regime. In regard to the Talmenes attack it said, 'The Leadership Panel is of the view that the Syrian Arab Forces used makeshift weapons deployed from helicopters, including those shaped like a barrel', and that the incident was the result of a 'Syrian Arab Armed Forces helicopter dropping a device causing damage to the structure of a concrete block building and was followed by the release of a toxic substance that affected the population'.

This was incredible. While the OPCW had previously declared that chemical weapons had been used in Syria, it had never before pointed the finger at the culprits. It was a real victory for Houssam and his colleagues. Their evidence had been key in showing the world that Assad was responsible for these attacks. Indeed, British Foreign Secretary Philip Hammond stated in response, 'The systematic and repeated use of chlorine in northern Syria and the consistent reports from witnesses of the presence of helicopters at the times of the attacks leave little doubt as to the Assad regime's culpability.'

However, to no one's great surprise, Russia and Syria again cried foul. The Russian Ambassador to the UK, Alexander Yakovenko, argued that the JIM was not only seriously flawed but also compromised by politicization. Once more, Russia used its UN veto to prevent action being taken, including the prevention of the sale of helicopters to the Syrian regime or even sanctions against Syrian commanders or officials linked to the attacks. Putin declared that such sanctions against Syria would be 'totally inappropriate'. Russia also blocked UN Security Council resolutions referring these crimes to the International Criminal Court, despite sixty other countries co-sponsoring them.

With the UN unable to take action, I wasn't under any illusions that the West would do so. After the previous humiliating loss in Parliament, the British Prime Minister, now Theresa May, would not risk a blow to her party's authority, particularly when it only had a limited majority and was preoccupied with Brexit.

Still, Houssam's evidence had set the ball rolling, making it clear for the first time since Syria became a signatory that Assad was in breach of the Chemical Weapons

Convention. In April 2018, as evidence against Assad continued to mount, a chlorine attack in Douma, where forty people died, finally provoked a response. With the OPCW confirming the results, which the Russians and the 'useful idiots' once more attempted to discredit, Parliament now voted to take action, without waiting for a UN Resolution.

The US, UK and France subsequently launched more than 100 missiles against a scientific research centre in Damascus, a chemical weapons storage facility west of Homs and another storage site and command post nearby. Announcing the launch, President Trump said the US was prepared to sustain economic, diplomatic and military pressure on Assad until he ended the use of chemical weapons. While I held out hope that this might deter Assad, it was made clear by US Secretary of Defense James Mattis that this was 'a one-time shot'. Sadly, this has proved to be the case. Despite all the evidence that Assad continues to use chemical weapons, the West has once again largely stood back.

However, though the situation in Syria continues to upset and appal, I am delighted to say that Houssam and his family are now safe and well. After being forced to flee their homeland. Houssam was awarded a scholarship at John Hopkins University in Baltimore, where he can finally finish his studies. He is one of a number of real heroes who have emerged from this terrible conflict. I know that he dreams of returning to Syria once he has qualified, to help rebuild his shattered and divided country. I am certain that, in time, the evidence he has collected will also ensure that Assad is convicted of war crimes.

As for me, I was still travelling to Bab al-Hawa Hospital in Syria to train medics, where I was soon to witness a scene that would shake me to my very core.

14

Harsh Reality

Things had been coming to a head for a long time, but at the end of 2014 the dam finally cracked.

It had become increasingly clear that, despite my best intentions, SecureBio wasn't working out. The cancellation of the Halabja project had hit us hard, but more importantly I found that my heart just wasn't in it. I loved working with the guys but I found office life stifling and frustrating. I had found a passion for helping doctors in Syria, but being away so often put a further strain on the business. We were just about keeping our heads above water but without someone to really drive the company forward, it was clear that was all we would ever do. And yet, even knowing that my heart wasn't in it, I couldn't just walk away. This was my only source of income. It was the only way I could afford to look after my family and keep making trips to Syria, which I funded myself. Something clearly had to give.

Thankfully, before I had to make a tough decision between SecureBio and Syria, an offer for the business came from out of the blue. Avon Rubber plc, a global leader in respiratory and ballistic protection for the world's militaries and first responders, wanted to buy us out. It would incorporate SecureBio into its business but would continue to employ Thommo, Olly and me (Rich had already moved on to a new job by this point). My title would be Managing Director of CBRN and the role would entail a whole host of responsibilities, not least adding some credibility with my first-hand experience of dealing with CBRN in war zones, which would certainly help when speaking to prospective clients. Though he was disappointed, and had lost money on SecureBio, my good friend Duckie graciously allowed the deal to go through. It was the only solution for us. The terms of the deal barely put us in profit, but the regular salary we would be paid as employees was a huge weight off my shoulders. I would no longer have to stress about making ends meet. For now, at least, I could try to find the best of both worlds. Putting in the required hours with Avon, I could still head off to Syria to help with sample collection and to train medical staff.

Bab al-Hawa Hospital was still the furthest I could reach in Syria, and I went there as often as I could, often meeting other Brits, who seemed to be performing miracles on a daily basis. One of these was Dr David Nott, who had been working on and off at the hospital and beyond for the last few years, using his NHS holiday allowance to come to Syria. Everyone spoke very highly of him but

I was still surprised to find just how nice and humble he was and is. David has saved the lives of countless people, and has also provided comfort to those who had no hope of survival. He has done all this with very limited medical equipment, staff and medicines. His ability to improvise under the most stressful situations is legendary. Even when all of the electricity and lighting went out in the hospital, he continued to operate. On one occasion, when everyone in the hospital was ordered to evacuate as it was thought the Syrian regime were preparing a strike, David continued to perform lifesaving surgery, knowing full well he could be killed at any moment.

Back in Britain, his influence has also been enormous. He has harangued Parliament and humanitarian organizations to do more, making a few enemies along the way with his refusal to compromise. He has done this for no reward, and it has come at a great cost, with David suffering from PTSD. If ever there is a man who deserves to be knighted, it is him.

We struck up a good relationship, and I was honoured when he asked me to work with him and the brilliant Dr Saleyah Ahsan on the Doctor's Under Fire initiative. We aimed to raise awareness, while also lobbying the Prime Minister to stop the Syrian regime from actively targeting doctors and hospitals.

As well as David, there was also James Le Mesurier, whom I had first met in Germany in 1999, where he was a fellow officer. He had struck me as a cheerful but committed man, dedicated to serving his country. In 2013, having left the military to work as an adviser on Syrian civil defence, he became appalled at the humanitarian crisis that was unfolding in the country. Determined to do something about it, he attempted to set up a full-time volunteer service to help those in need.

Syrians and foreigners flocked to the cause and were the first to rush in to help victims when bombs rained down. In doing so, they risked their lives to help anyone in need, regardless of religion or politics, while also pledging allegiance to a set of international humanitarian values and principles as laid out in the Geneva Conventions.

Known as the 'White Helmets', owing to their uniforms, most of these men and women were not medical professionals. They were decorators, taxi drivers, bakers, tailors, engineers, pharmacists, shopkeepers, painters, carpenters, students and even housewives, a truly disparate mix of people with one common goal: to save lives. And they have: over 100,000 lives have been saved since the White Helmets were founded. However, many volunteers have paid the ultimate price for their compassion, with hundreds of men and women killed while saving others. As James said in an August 2015 interview:

'They are all a very diverse and disparate group of individuals, all of whom made individual choices . . . They all had the choice whether or not they want to pick up a gun, to become a refugee – but they've all made a choice to instead pick up a stretcher.'

The White Helmets' motto is taken from the Quran: 'To save a life is to save all of humanity.' I cannot think of anything more appropriate.

However, as matters escalated, the White Helmets soon became targets themselves. As I said previously, Assad's strategy was not to just fight rebels on the battlefield but also to kill anyone who might be helping them, as well as to destroy all associated infrastructure. The decimation of medical services was central to this strategy. As such, hospitals, clinics, drug warehouses and blood banks were systematically targeted, as well as the White Helmets. 'Double tap' attacks became routine: the Syrian regime would first target a civilian population and then return to kill the White Helmets who were rushing in to help the wounded.

Having got the ball rolling on the White Helmets, simultaneously setting up an ambulance, fire and medical service in Syria, James asked for my support after the 2013 attack in Ghouta. Many White Helmets had died of cross contamination when treating patients, and James asked if I could help train them. Our paths would cross many times after this, and we would occasionally meet for a coffee at his Istanbul HQ to discuss the crisis.

One afternoon, as I spoke to a room full of doctors in Bab al-Hawa, I saw first-hand why David and James's

White Helmets organization was so highly valued, as the hospital suddenly came alive with shouts and piercing screams. Breaking away from the room, I looked out into the corridor to be confronted by pandemonium. Amongst a cacophony of noise, men, women and children of all ages were being dumped against the walls by overworked White Helmet paramedics. With the smell of burning flesh in my nostrils, I looked on in shock as temporary tourniquets were tied to shattered arms and legs. There was no time to waste, and some surgeons were already operating on the floor, amputating the remains of bloodied limbs and hurriedly administering morphine to try to dull the excruciating pain. In a daze, I looked around: there were people with half their heads missing or their buttocks blown off. On the floor before me was a pool of blood, pumping from a woman's exposed pulmonary artery. Her glazed eyes and pale skin told me she did not have long to live. As the screams and shouts reverberated around my head, I felt physically and emotionally sick. I had seen many colleagues injured or killed in action, but this was the first time I had really seen the devastation that war could wreak on innocent civilians.

Shortly before, a Syrian regime helicopter had apparently dropped a large steel drum, packed with 500 kilograms of TNT, on to a playground in Aleppo, the supposed hiding place of a terrorist. To the regime it did not matter that children were playing there; their lives were expendable in the quest to destroy all opposition. The effect of these so-called barrel bombs was catastrophic, decimating the body on impact or shredding its skin and organs with shrapnel. Seeing these injuries in the flesh was horrifying. I felt totally powerless as ambulance after ambulance continued to pull up outside. Thankfully, Dr David Nott emerged to take control of the situation.

As I watched him in action for the first time, quickly checking on the most injured, calming screaming children and shouting out orders to prepare the operating theatre, I was in awe. Somehow, he managed to keep a calm head while operating at an incredibly high level. This was a set of skills I had only ever seen a handful of times in my life. It was truly extraordinary. And alongside David, moving in and out of the corridor, were White Helmet paramedics, their white uniforms now speckled with blood.

Watching the White Helmets carry in the wounded on stretchers while David and his doctors tended to them made me momentarily proud to be British. While the world had turned its back on Syria, David and James were risking their lives, expecting nothing in return, to help save the lives of people of different colours, creeds and religions.

Yet other fleeting thoughts also crossed my mind in the middle of the horrific scene: how could human beings be so cruel to each other? Many of these poor innocent souls were children. How could someone like Assad, who has children of his own, give such an order? What did the helicopter pilot think before dropping the bomb, knowing that down below was a playground full of children trying to find a moment's happiness in a war zone? How could they sleep at night?

Watching the carnage unfold around me felt like a lifetime but it must have lasted a matter of minutes at most. All I could do, when I did manage to gather my senses, was to stumble back to the room where I had been holding the seminar. The doctors I had been teaching all stared at me as I struggled to find the words, my senses jumbled. 'I . . . uh, I will have to cancel the class, I'm afraid, so that you can . . . uh, help.' However, as I stood there, shaken to my core, I was surprised by their response.

'Hamish, we have plenty of doctors who can treat these conventional injuries,' one of them said. 'But we need to know about the gas. That is what really concerns us. We can hide from bombs and bullets but not gas.' Despite the total devastation I had just witnessed it was still chemical weapons that scared Syrians more than anything else.

Somehow, with all of the commotion continuing outside, and with my head ringing, we continued the class. But as I spoke, a strange sensation crept over me. I felt numb, as if it wasn't really me talking, almost like an out-of-body experience. It was as if I had just watched a movie and I wasn't really present. I somehow managed to finish the class but I almost couldn't remember a thing about it. It was as if I had been on autopilot.

As planned, after the seminar I made my way back to the border, where I would stay in my hotel on the Turkish side and return to the hospital the next day. Travelling through the remnants of destroyed towns, our car bouncing over the war-torn roads, I suddenly felt exhausted. I couldn't wait to get to my hotel, have a warm bath and get into bed, which instantly made me feel guilty as we passed families rooting through the ruins of their devastated homes.

Reaching the border in the early evening, we joined a queue of vehicles that were being inspected by the guards before being allowed to cross. Just in front of us was a White Helmet ambulance, its driver embroiled in an esca-lating argument with one of the guards. It appeared that he did not have the correct paperwork and I was momentarily angry that he was holding us all up.

Yet as we watched the guard refusing to give the ambulance permission to cross, the driver leapt out of the vehicle and marched to the back door. Swinging it open, he pointed to his cargo and made a last-ditch desperate appeal for mercy. Leaning forward, I squinted my eyes so that I could see through our dusty windscreen. In the back of the ambulance was a girl, no more than eight years old, with all of her limbs missing. I now understood the urgency. This girl needed urgent treatment in a better-equipped Turkish hospital or she would die.

For just a split second my eyes caught hers. It was like a shot through my heart. I could see she was scared. In an instant, all the numbness I had been feeling had been washed away only to be replaced by searing pain. This poor girl was being left to die alone, with not a single family member to comfort her. Because she was Syrian, the world had decided she wasn't worth saving. She couldn't even cross a border to reach a hospital where she might be able to get treatment.

I jumped out of the truck. I had no idea what I could do but my body had made the decision before my brain could react.

'Please,' I said, no doubt repeating the words the driver had been saying over and over. 'You have to let her cross! Please!'

At this the guard barked in my direction, 'Get back in your vehicle! Get back in your vehicle!'

'She's dying!' I spluttered, unable to comprehend how anyone could turn this little girl away, whatever laws and regulations they were supposed to adhere to.

But again, this cut no ice. 'Back! Now! Or you will be arrested.'

I pulled out my phone, intending to call Dr Ghanem to see if he knew anyone who could help. But as I did so, I noticed the driver had stopped his pleading. Looking towards the ambulance, I suddenly understood why. There was no need. The little girl had passed away. Her frozen eyes stared up at the ceiling, specks of blood splattered across her porcelain cheeks. Now all that remained was to cover her body with a white sheet.

No one even knew her name. Her future had been cruelly snatched away without so much as a thought. Just another statistic, another body to be dumped in a mass grave like a piece of rubbish. If her parents were still alive, they might not even know their daughter's fate. As I stared at what had once been a beautiful, smiling face, I almost couldn't process what I had seen. Days later, I finally cracked.

15

Breakdown and Breakthrough

After everything I had seen, I was relieved to get home and spend some time with my family. It was time to decompress and try to find some sense of normality. After my initial blip following the first Gulf War, I had learnt over time how to manage this, taking a few days out before throwing myself back into normal life. That usually did the trick and allowed me to adjust to a different pace. But now things felt different.

For a few weeks, I had found myself feeling ever more detached, as if life was going in slow motion and I was looking down on myself from above. I wasn't taking any medication but I felt foggy, as if a black cloud was hanging over me. In the past, some hard physical exercise had always got me out of a slump, but even this didn't interest me. I found myself lying in bed longer, rather than jumping out at the crack of dawn, eager to see what the day would bring. Emails and phone calls were also going unanswered, as I felt a growing sense of detachment from the world. If

I thought about Syria, it felt as if spiders were crawling up my skin. I had to physically shake myself to snap out of it. However, I kept such thoughts to myself and hoped that in time all this would pass.

Meanwhile, Julia became concerned that our beloved Labrador, Butler, seemed lethargic and had lost his appetite. As his weight plummeted, I took him to the vet, where our worst fears were confirmed. It was cancer and there was no hope. I had been in this position before with family pets, and while it was always sad, it had never really affected me in the way it did now. On this occasion, stroking Butler's fur and looking into his dying eyes as the vet administered the lethal injection, I struggled to compose myself. *Pull yourself together,* I thought. *You've been in a war zone for weeks and didn't react like this.* Yet the look in Butler's eyes, as his life ebbed away, was all too familiar. Images of the little girl on the Syrian border flashed into my mind.

As I took Butler to his favourite field and began to dig a hole in which to bury him, something broke inside me. Staring at his lifeless body, tears suddenly streaked down my face while my chest heaved, making it difficult to breathe. I couldn't control myself. It was as if a dam had burst and nothing would plug it. I had never experienced anything like it.

My upbringing – my father, boarding school, the army – had taught me to bottle things up. Reaching out for help wasn't an option, and there was certainly no time for emotions in a war zone. I was trained to be a macho soldier, and to do my job, come what may. While many of my colleagues had been treated for PTSD over the years, I had thought that maybe that part of my brain was missing or perhaps I was tougher than most. Deep down, I also had this insane view that perhaps those who suffered from PTSD weren't made of stern enough stuff. We all knew the job could be gruesome and bloody, so just got on with it.

This frame of mind had also seeped into my home life. Julia had always remarked that I could be quite cold at times and struggled with showing emotion or affection. But this was merely a coping mechanism that had been drummed into me from a young age and had seen me through some pretty horrific times, not least my experience in the Gulf. If I let my guard down for a moment, I feared I would not be as effective on the battlefield, where my life was at risk. Now it seemed I had reached my limit, as if a dormant volcano had finally blown its top.

It took more than six hours to dig the hole, most of which I sat beside it sobbing. The image of that poor little girl, stranded in the ambulance at the border, her life slowly slipping away when she could have been saved, tore into me. No rubbish about putting on a brave face could stop my gut-wrenching flood of tears.

That evening, looking bereft with my eyes red raw, Julia could tell that all was not well. She had never seen me like this before, and it was clear this went way beyond the death of a beloved family pet. 'You can talk to me, Hamish, you know,' Julia said. 'I know you've seen things you don't like to talk about but I'm here for you.' Perhaps for the first time in our entire relationship I suddenly opened up, and I couldn't stop.

Taking a seat, I told Julia for the first time about the scenes in the hospital, then the bombs, the chemicals, the cities razed to the ground, the thousands of maimed children, families with nowhere to go, surrounded by war and famine at every turn, and then, finally, the fate of that little girl. 'They just left her to die,' I spluttered angrily. Holding my hand as this torrent of inhumanity poured out of me, Julia said, 'Hamish, do you think you need to see someone?'

The thought of speaking about such things with a stranger was abhorrent to me. I was ashamed to be speaking about them with my wife, let alone with someone who didn't know me. It was something that just didn't sit right with me, but over the next few days Julia was insistent. She showed me countless articles in which other military personnel, who were certainly far tougher than I was, extolled the virtues of counselling. But though I was slowly coming around to the idea, I just couldn't follow through and make an appointment.

Julia soon took matters into her own hands. 'Hamish,' she announced matter-of-factly, 'I've made you an appointment with a counsellor for 10 a.m. on Friday. I'll drive you there.' This was, of course, to ensure that I actually went, but I said there was no need and drove myself.

Now what I say next is not how these stories are meant to go. I'm meant to say I went for counselling and emerged a new and enlightened man. I'm meant to now be a role model for speaking out about my mental health and describe how talking to a counsellor changed my life. But the thing is, it didn't. The more I spoke about my experiences the more it just felt like self-pity, when I was very well aware that millions of Syrians were suffering far worse than I was. If anything, talking about Syria just made me angrier than I was before. I became consumed with rage at how this was all being allowed to happen, with those in power knowing full well the atrocities that were being committed. Millions of people were being displaced from their homes and allowed to perish, all to keep one man in power.

To be honest, my poor counsellor never stood much of a chance. I went in with a negative attitude and left with it. If I had been more open to the experience, I might have found the many benefits that so many people speak about. And I certainly have not discounted going back again, as the results speak for themselves. It just didn't feel like, at that time in my life, it was something that was going to help me.

The war in Syria was intensifying. Every hour I sat in that chair talking, I felt I could have been out there actually making some sort of difference. So, once more, I packed all of my emotions into a box and buried them deep, ready to be unboxed at another, more convenient time, if there is such a thing. But what I did have was a new-found determination to help. It was the only thing that would keep me going. In a roundabout way, the counselling session had at least awakened this within me and allowed me to chart a way forward.

During this period, I had kept in contact with people I had met in Syria, most notably David Nott and James Le Mesurier. In early December 2016, David told me that conditions in Aleppo were worsening, which was hard to imagine, as on my last visit things had already been pretty grim.

Ever since the FSA had taken control of most of Syria's most populous city in 2012, there had been a stalemate. However, in the summer of 2015, with Assad believed to be losing the war, Russia and Iran came to the rescue, supplying warplanes, attack helicopters, artillery pieces, military advisers and battle-hardened fighters. This support quickly turned the tide. By September 2015 Assad's forces were strong enough to launch a concerted effort to seize Aleppo. By December they had made significant advances around the city and by February 2016 had nearly surrounded it. When Russian air strikes helped close the rebels' last supply line in July 2016, a five-month siege began, known to many as 'Syria's Stalingrad'.

Breakdown and Breakthrough

Assad and his allies imposed a blockade on rebel areas, cutting off supplies to some 320,000 people. The rebels briefly broke the siege, but Assad's forces quickly reimposed it, unleashing wave after wave of ferocious bombardments. Nothing and no one was spared. As we know all too well by now, women and children were fair game, as were hospitals, schools and heritage sites. Even children's hospitals were bombed. As Assad saw it, while there were many innocents in the city there were also many enemies. By levelling it, he would at least ensure that his enemies had been crushed, no matter how many war crimes he had to commit to do so.

The UN High Commissioner for Human Rights, Sir Stephen O'Brien, warned that 'crimes of historic proportions' were being committed but, again, the UN, and the world at large, had made its choice. Getting bogged down in the quagmire of Syria was just too risky. Grand speeches by politicians expressing shock and outrage were par for the course but the Syrian people now needed far more than words of condemnation. But no one was willing to ride to the rescue. Aleppo and its people had been abandoned.

David told me that things now looked to be coming to a horrific close, after four years of fighting and one of the longest sieges in modern warfare. The Syrian regime had begun dropping leaflets on the city which read: 'If you do not leave these areas urgently, you will be annihilated . . . You know that everyone has given up on you. They left

231

you alone to face your doom and nobody will give you any help.' With these chilling words, it was clear that Assad was planning to put an end to this once and for all.

David also told me that while most were trying to leave the city there were hundreds of children who had been seriously injured in the attacks who were unable to do so. Many of them were amputees, paraplegics or worse. Some were orphans, having lost their families in the war. As the city emptied, they were effectively being left to die alone. Something drastic needed to be done.

At the time David was still working regularly at the Bab al-Hawa Hospital. We reasoned that if we could somehow get the children out of Aleppo and to David's hospital we would at least save them from the coming bombardment. For me, it also offered the chance of redemption. Having felt powerless and been left bereft as the little girl had died at the border, there was now something I could do to help hundreds of others. In my head at least, this would ensure that her tragic death had not been in vain. But it would not be easy.

With the air strikes scheduled to hit imminently, we couldn't risk taking sick children out in such an environment. Somehow we needed to get Assad and Putin to call a ceasefire for a few hours. This seemed a ridiculous proposition but, by a miraculous chain of events, David had actually met Assad many years before, when he had worked as an ophthalmic surgeon in London in the 1990s.

That was before his elder brother, Bassel, who had been earmarked to rule Syria following their father, died in a car crash in 1994. From that moment Assad's medical career had been cut short and his rise to bloodthirsty dictator had begun. Though David no longer had a direct line to Assad, he knew others who could help him reach the president.

On receiving a number to call, David made first contact on 7 December. Speaking to an intermediary, David was not sure if Assad himself was actually present on the call, but was told he would receive any message. In any event, David outlined the desperate situation and pleaded for a ceasefire so that we could evacuate the sick children. While his plea for a ceasefire was not dismissed out of hand, neither was any commitment forthcoming. The only thing the intermediary muttered was, 'No UN buses can be used to transport the children. Syrian regime buses only.' This seemed to suggest an opening. There was at least hope.

Meanwhile, conditions in Aleppo worsened. Barrel bombs containing chlorine had been dropped, while hundreds of men were reported missing after crossing from rebel-held areas of Aleppo into government territory. The only area of Aleppo not yet controlled by Assad had shrunk to just two or three square kilometres, where over 100,000 people were trapped, while there were reports that the rebels were preventing people from leaving, in order to use them as human shields.

As the temperature had dropped to minus ten, and the

decimated city was battered by blizzards, civilians were expected to be able to hold out for only five more days, with food and medicine scarce. We also learnt that many of the children we had hoped to save were dying. At this David and I increased our efforts, calling everyone we knew who held any semblance of power in the UK and the US to ask for help, while also speaking to Assad's intermediary every day, hoping for a chink of light. However, complicating matters was the news that a Russian field hospital in west Aleppo had been shelled by the rebels and two Russian doctors had died. Now we were being told that there were catastrophes on both sides and that was the cost of war, as if the lives of hundreds of innocent children did not matter.

As the MP Andrew Mitchell chaired an emergency debate in the House of Commons, David finally made a breakthrough. A contact had managed to discuss the situation with the Russian government. Soon after, David received a call from a withheld number. It was Putin himself. Unphased, David calmly asked for a 24-hour ceasefire so that we could get the children out of the city on humanitarian grounds. Putin did not yet commit, but his final words to David were somewhat ominous: 'Tell your friend de Bretton-Gordon to stop accusing Assad of chemical attacks.'

I took this to be a threat, particularly as I had been regularly receiving death threats on social media from Russian bot accounts. Nevertheless, soon after this we heard some promising news. A ceasefire was to come into force from all sides, and the regime would supply a convoy of green buses to ferry the children out. I could not believe it, but it seemed to be happening. However, despite the good news about the ceasefire, there were still some legitimate concerns.

The Russians and the Syrian regime manned all the routes out of the city. Despite assurances, there was no guarantee that those leaving wouldn't be killed or arrested on the way to Bab al-Hawa. Indeed, a few weeks previously, a UN convoy, delivering medical aid and food into east Aleppo, had come under attack from the air and was wiped out, even though its presence had been agreed by the Syrian regime. Both the Russian and Syrian air forces denied responsibility, which was laughable. Yet, in these perilous circumstances, we had no option but to take the Russians and Syrians at their word, something which didn't sit easily with anyone.

By now temperatures in Aleppo had plummeted, with ice and snow making conditions treacherous. As the green buses struggled to reach the hospital, the children and their carers waited outside. Tragically, before the operation had even got underway, three babies froze to death. It was a devastating blow. When the green buses finally arrived, the children were loaded on board. With no time to waste before the bombing resumed, they desperately worked their way through the rubble, ice and snow to get out of the city and reach a crossing point, where they were handed over to Syria Relief, whose ambulances would take the sick and wounded to the hospital in Bab al-Hawa.

While they soon arrived at the hospital, and in good time, considering the circumstances, without any trouble from the regime or Russians, David was dismayed to find that some of the children were in a worse state than he had feared, especially after travelling in the cold and in buses not particularly suited to their medical needs. It became apparent to David and the other doctors that many of the children required urgent operations if they were going to survive. This was where I now came in.

While David had been tirelessly helping to negotiate the ceasefire, I had also been hard at work. As word went around about our proposed mission, we had received offers of support from the most incredible places. Sir Bob Geldof was keen to do all he could, as was the entrepreneur Rory McCarthy. Yet the most vital offer came from Virgin Atlantic boss Sir Richard Branson, who promised to lend us a plane on Christmas Eve to get the children to Britain. However, there was a slight snag: we would only have it for twelve hours as it was then due to go to Alicante. It was a very tight time frame but it was certainly achievable – if everything went like clockwork. On hearing of this, the Health Secretary Jeremy Hunt told us, 'If you can get the children to Britain, I will ensure they can be treated on the NHS.' This seemed a tremendous opportunity. In

Britain they would not only escape a war zone but would also be properly treated. But getting hundreds of poorly children to Britain, in the lead-up to Christmas, was going to be a significant challenge.

While we had the Virgin plane on loan for only twelve hours, other issues were mounting. A Virgin pilot's strike was being threatened over Christmas, which would leave us without a pilot or crew. Worse still, the local airport we planned to use near the border was not licensed for UK aircraft. As I tried to rectify this, it suddenly struck me that we had an even bigger problem to contend with.

We had initially thought that the plane would be big enough to carry all of the children. However, we had not factored in that many of them were desperately ill and would need rows to themselves, as well as seats for their carers. This required making some tough decisions. Only the worst-off children, who would most benefit from NHS treatment, would be able to fly. And they would have to leave any parents behind, so that we could fit as many of them on the plane as possible. This was far from ideal, but in testing circumstances, and with time getting away from us, it seemed the only option we had. But this presented yet another issue: many of the children did not have passports of their own.

Back at home in Salisbury I worked frantically to resolve these situations. Since it was Christmas, Julia and the kids weren't too amused to find I wouldn't be able to join in all things jolly until the situation had been resolved. However, when I told them what was going on, they were tremendously supportive, particularly as everything was being held together by such slender threads. Tempers were also fraying amongst those who had been trying to help. The combination of it being the lead-up to Christmas and having such limited time available tested the best of us. There were quite a few angry conversations and phones slammed down, which wasn't quite in keeping with the festive spirit, but all everyone wanted was for the children to be safe and well.

As Christmas Eve arrived, I had worked 24/7 to get everything in order. The NHS hospitals were on standby, the passport situation had been resolved, the plane was on the runway, fully staffed, but there was one thing outstanding. No matter where I turned, I could not get the flight plan approved. Things were now getting desperate. With time ticking before we would lose the plane to its Alicante slot, I was becoming increasingly stressed when David called. Having by now had a chance to operate on many of the children and stabilize others, he wasn't sure if many of them would actually benefit from coming to the UK. Some were sadly beyond help. All he could do was make them as comfortable as they could be. Others would be better off remaining with their families while they recovered. He felt that there were only five children who could receive better care elsewhere than he could currently provide, and that he could arrange for them to receive that in Turkey, where their parents could join them.

In testing circumstances, this seemed the best option. It was perhaps not the Christmas miracle we had envisaged, and I know a number of people in the UK were bitterly disappointed that all their hard work had come to nothing, but the reason we were doing all of this was for the children, and they were safe.

As I sat down for Christmas Day with my family, while I had not entirely shifted the emotional gloom that had previously rocked me so hard, I did find some peace in knowing that I had played a small part in ensuring that many children had escaped further atrocities. Yet I also spared a thought for all those who were not so lucky.

When the ceasefire ended, Aleppo was razed to the ground, leaving just a wasteland of flattened buildings, concrete rubble and bullet-pocked walls where once hundreds of thousands of people had lived. Although the rebels and civilians had surrendered, that still did not stop them from being tortured and executed. The best they could hope for was prison or conscription.

As the world's worst refugee crisis unfolded, US Ambassador to the UN Samantha Power said, 'Aleppo will join the ranks of those events in world history that define modern evil, that stain our conscience decades later – Halabja, Rwanda, Srebrenica and now Aleppo.'

However, the war was not yet over, and as such David

and I were still determined to continue our work. A year later, and after learning some vital lessons, we again negotiated a ceasefire and managed to evacuate thirty-two children who were suffering from cancer out of Ghouta and on to Damascus, where they could be treated by the International Red Crescent. I'm very happy to say that, as far as I am aware, all of those children were successfully treated and survived.

I might not know the name of the little girl who died in the back of the ambulance on the border but her life was not lost in vain. She inspired me, and in turns others, to save the lives of other children, just like her. Until my dying day, I'll never forget her.

Part Three

'On Innocent Tongues'

16

Full Circle

It was still a deep regret of mine that the Halabja project had been postponed due to the rise of ISIS. I had really warmed to the Kurdish people and was keen to help them. While it didn't look like the project would be resurrected any time soon, an opportunity soon presented itself that could not only help the Kurds but also lay some of my personal ghosts to rest.

By December 2015 ISIS held a large area extending from western Iraq to eastern Syria, containing an estimated 8 to 12 million people. With its brutal interpretation of Sharia law being enforced within these borders, anyone who stood in the terror group's way could expect to be dealt with mercilessly. Videos soon circulated the globe of enemy fighters being beheaded, hanged, burnt alive or stoned to death. With an estimated annual budget of more than $1 billion and a force of more than 30,000 fighters, ISIS was a force to be reckoned with, especially when it managed to obtain chemical weapons.

After the Gulf War, the UN had buried some of Saddam's chemical stockpile in a concrete bunker at Al Muthanna, just outside Baghdad. The stockpile included 2,500 degraded chemical rockets filled with sarin, about 180 tonnes of sodium cyanide, a very toxic chemical that was a precursor for the nerve agent tabun, 2,000 empty 155mm artillery shells contaminated with mustard gas, 605 one-tonne mustard gas containers with residues, as well as heavily contaminated construction material. In 2014, as the country again spiralled out of control and guards fled the site, ISIS fighters ram-raided Al Muthanna and made off with whatever they could lay their hands on.

Some suggested that by this stage the chemicals from Al Muthanna would have been sufficiently degraded to not be any danger. It is therefore difficult to say whether or not ISIS was able to deploy them, but what is undeniable is that soon afterwards it launched a number of chemical attacks throughout Syria and Iraq. Indeed, a study released by IHS Conflict Monitor, a London-based intelligence collection and analysis service, claimed that by 2016 the group had used chlorine and mustard gas at least fifty-two times in the region. Once more, it was the Kurds in northern Iraq who would suffer the most, as ISIS looked to turn Kurdistan into a caliphate.

The first attack came on 11 August 2015, when a village south of the capital, Erbil, was hit by fifty mortar rounds of chlorine. With no protective equipment, gas masks or training, the Kurdish civilians and Peshmerga fighters didn't stand a chance. Almost immediately, forty men, women and children became sick, with burning eyes and lungs, and painful blisters erupting all over their bodies. In the months that followed, chlorine and mustard gas were hurtled at Peshmerga troops in further attacks via canisters, grenades, mortar shells and even artillery rockets.

The rise in these chemical attacks prompted the Kurdish regional government to issue an urgent plea for gas masks to Washington and other Western capitals. Without them the Kurds were sitting ducks. But once more the West was slow to offer help. However, at this time I was actually in Baghdad, through my job with Avon, working on a potential deal to sell gas marks to the Iraqi military.

After many previous visits I knew my way around Baghdad, but this occasion felt different. With ISIS at the gates, everyone was on edge. The Iraqi Army had just capitulated in Ramadi, Kirkuk and Mosul and ISIS's march into Baghdad felt inevitable. It was clear that the enemy was also growing from within. You could feel the tension every time you stepped outside. No one was to be trusted, even more so than usual. I was therefore relieved to be staying in the relative safety of the British Embassy in the Green Zone, a walled compound for coalition forces in the centre of Baghdad. While not five-star standard by any means, I had a comfortable room, as well as a decent gym and pool, and a hotel bar that I could frequent to let off some steam. In such circumstances, this was a luxury.

As I said, the goal of my trip was to sell gas masks from Avon to the Iraqi military. Yet while the Iraqi military did indeed desperately require gas masks, its representatives were only looking to do business with people who were prepared to oil the wheels. Shortly after I had arrived, I found that a Chinese rival had handed over $500,000 to those in charge and subsequently secured the $32m contract. This was a bit of a blow but I'm certainly glad we refused to get involved in any nonsense like that, as not long after those involved in the deal were charged with corruption and either jailed or shot. The Iraqi Army did not get their masks either. It seemed it was a bad deal all round, but certainly nothing out of the ordinary in the Wild West of Baghdad at that time.

The trip looked like a total bust, and I was preparing to make my way home when I learnt of the Kurds' plea for gas masks. After my work on the grave sites in Halabja, I had kept in contact with many of my Kurdish friends, especially Shwan Zulal, a London-based journalist who had helped us on the Halabja project, and I had developed a deep respect for them. If they needed gas masks, I was determined to help.

I realized that Avon had a number of escape hoods that only had a two-year shelf life. This was too short a period for most armies, who wanted a five-year certification, so Avon was unable to sell them. I managed to convince the then CEO, a compassionate chap called Rob Rennie, who sadly did not last long in his post, that we should give the hoods, as a humanitarian gesture, to the Peshmerga. He agreed to let me have five hundred of them, and soon after they were shipped to Erbil. But I knew this still wouldn't be enough. For them to really be effective, I had to train the Peshmerga how to use them, as well as how to combat chemical weapons.

On my previous visits to Kurdistan, I had got to know Brigadier Hajar, the Peshmerga's main CBRN man. After making a phone call, the Brigadier told me that most of the chemical attacks were in Sector 6, just east of Mosul, with a front line of about 100 kilometres. With its proximity to Erbil, home to two million people, it was of the highest strategic importance. ISIS had already got to within 10 kilometres of the capital and though the Peshmerga pushed them all the way back to Gwer, and then across the river to Mosul, they were now regrouping and ramping up their use of chemical weapons. He therefore urgently organized the escape hoods' onward transit to the front line and made arrangements for me to visit.

Despite the threat from ISIS, I found the atmosphere in Erbil far more relaxed than in Baghdad. Having been greeted at the airport by officers of the Peshmerga Black

Panther division, who were tasked with defending Erbil, I was taken in their white Toyota pickup, with its Black Panther emblem emblazoned on the bonnet, to the beautiful five-star Rotana Hotel, which was as lovely as any place in the world. In such luxury I suddenly felt very tranquil, as if I was on a holiday rather than preparing a military unit to face one of the most murderous terror groups the world has ever known. It had a great gym and pool, while the top two floors were given over to the British Consulate, which made me feel even more at home.

Waking early the next day, I was transported to the Black Panthers' HQ, which was just 1,500 metres behind the front line at Gwer. Colonel Srud Bazarni, the sector's Chief of Staff and a very impressive officer, had gathered about one hundred of his men inside a large tent. It was blisteringly hot, and there was no air conditioning, but no one flinched. Everyone was eager to learn, especially as there had been a mustard gas attack the day before and a chlorine attack the day before that. Minds were very much focused. Most of the soldiers there would have been affected in some way by the chemical attacks in the late 1980s and many feared this fate now befalling them and their families.

Knowing the impact of these attacks, I immediately tried to settle their nerves. I still remembered how it felt to be terrified of chemical weapons, and I wanted them to understand that most could be easily combatted. 'Chlorine or mustard gas can only kill you if you swallow it or breathe it in,' I said via a translator. Now holding up an escape hood, I continued: 'If you wear these, the gas cannot kill you.' At this I proceeded to hand out the escape hoods, apparently to some bemusement.

'Hamish, we have a problem with your escape hoods,' one of the young officers said, an articulate captain who, I learnt, had completed the elite US Ranger course.

'OK,' I replied. 'What is it?'

'We cannot use them – the Peshmerga never escape. We fight to the death,'

I knew this to be true, so I answered, 'If we just call them hoods, will that cover it?'

'Yes, that covers it nicely,' he smiled in return.

I went on to explain that the soldiers should try to know which way the wind was blowing, because the chemicals will always be blown downwind. Hence in a chemical attack you should run as fast as you can across the wind, or get to higher ground, as the gas, heavier than air, quickly sinks to the lowest areas.

Again, the officer put up his hand. 'Hamish, we can't do this,' he declared. 'The Peshmerga never run away!'

I smiled. I had not thought of this either. 'How about you relocate as quickly as you can?' I suggested.

'Yes, we can do that!' he answered, seemingly satisfied that the Peshmerga's bravery would not be compromised.

With the training at an end, and the soldiers satisfied that the escape hoods could be useful, Colonel Srud suggested we conduct a tour of the front line. With the officers in tow, we duly drove due west towards Mosul and stopped at the major river crossing at Gwer. Again, the scenery was stunning. As lots of Peshmerga officers and vehicles moved to and fro from the small Kurdish town behind us, we stood at the edge of the river raging below, which was glimmering in the sunshine. I saw that the bridge crossing the river had recently been blown to stop ISIS from crossing, and its crippled steel remnants could still be seen scattered across the water.

I was still admiring the scenery when I suddenly heard the crack of sniper fire in the distance. I momentarily flinched before another sound caught my attention . . .

Thump! Thump! Thump!

Wincing into the sun, I saw mortars being fired at us from ISIS positions across the river. As the mortars hit the ground, I braced myself for an explosion but I instead heard a 'pop'. Immediately I knew these must be chemical weapons. The 'pop' sound was the detonator splitting the shell case to release the chemical. A cloud of green and yellow chlorine gas quickly dispersed, the wind carrying it towards us. My mind instantly flashed back to the all-consuming panic I had felt when supposedly under attack in the Gulf War over two decades before. But a lot had changed since then. Rather than feeling terrified, as I had

250

been in 1991, I knew that this was my chance to demonstrate that this was actually a psychological weapon as much a physical one, not only to the Peshmerga but also to myself.

'Put on your hoods!' I shouted, as more mortars were fired in our direction.

Thump! Thump! Thump!

Everyone hurriedly put on their hoods and I shouted to them to follow me as more gas dispersed, blowing ominously towards us. Some were hesitant but as I was leading the way and seemed to be breathing freely, they quickly joined me, racing towards the gas instead of away from it.

Approaching the mortars before some had a chance to detonate, I saw that they were 122mm in diameter with perhaps two litres of chlorine inside. Suddenly I saw a real change come over the men. They were standing in the middle of the gas, totally unharmed. Watching them, it seemed that a barrier in their minds had now been lifted. Rather than being on the defensive, they were now ready to attack.

As a drone approached from the ISIS position, whizzing above our heads, conducting a damage assessment, the Peshmerga loosed off everything they had at it to bring it down. Then they charged forwards, shooting and shouting, showing that they were unafraid. It was a remarkable sight. Never before had I seen such an instant change come over so many people. The fear of chemical weapons was gone.

A French military team arrived at the front line later in the day and, after inspecting the site, they confirmed a chlorine attack had taken place. It seemed that the Peshmerga had received their escape hoods just in time. As I bid General Bazarni and his men farewell, I felt proud of my relationship with the Kurds and that I had been able to offer some assistance. For more than a generation, the Kurds have known only war, first with Saddam Hussein and then with ISIS. But just as was the case with Saddam, the Kurds in Iraq once more prevailed, finally defeating ISIS in 2017. I hope that one day we might even be able to complete the Halabja project, which I am sure will allow a lot of families to finally be able to begin the healing process.

The Kurds had prevailed, and the incident had also allowed me to banish some ghosts of my past. It had been over twenty-five years since the incident in the Gulf, and it had marked my life ever since. Even as I had grown more confident and accomplished in dealing with chemical and biological weapons, it was always in the back of my mind. I had done many things in my career since but I had not yet been in the middle of an actual chemical attack. I had often wondered how I would react, knowing just how scared I had been the first time around. The fact that I was now able to run towards an attack, rather than away from one, was a real accomplishment. I felt as if a psychological load had suddenly been lifted and there was nothing now left for me to fear. But while that load had been lifted, and I looked to the future with a new confidence, the world soon faced a new threat, as chemical attacks were seen outside Syria, with even my home town, Salisbury, coming under attack.

17

Salisbury

In March 2018, I delivered the keynote speech at the Abu Dhabi International Defence Show, speaking primarily about the threat of home soil attacks. Intelligence reports suggested that a terror group, such as ISIS, were now looking to attack the West. Indeed, there were signs that despots had already taken the West's inaction against Assad as a green light to use chemical weapons as they saw fit.

On 13 February 2017, Kim Jong-nam, the half-brother of the North Korean leader Kim Jong-un, had arrived at Kuala Lumpur's international airport to catch a flight to Macau. He had recently fallen foul of his infamous sibling and it was also known that he had been working for the CIA, so he had to have his wits about him.

With a backpack slung over his shoulder, he marched through the hectic airport and looked for the check-in desk. Meanwhile, CCTV footage picked up a woman watching his every move. Suddenly, with his attention averted, she jumped in front of him and wiped a cloth covered in an oily substance over his face, while another woman grabbed him from behind and covered his eyes with her hands. As Kim brushed them off, no doubt fearing for his life, they quickly fled.

Immediately feeling dizzy, Kim complained to customer services about the incident but collapsed soon after. Rushed to hospital, he was given a 1mg shot of atropine and a shot of adrenalin, but it was no use. Less than twenty minutes after the attack Kim Jong-nam was dead, the victim of an assassination carried out with the nerve agent VX, one of the deadliest chemical weapons in the world.

It transpired soon after that four North Korean suspects had left the airport after the assassination and had fled to Pyongyang. However, the two women who had actually carried out the attack were arrested and found to be former escorts from Indonesia and Vietnam. According to their testimonies, in the previous months the women had been unknowingly groomed as killers by North Korean agents and had thought they were carrying out a prank for a Japanese YouTube show. I found this difficult to believe, particularly as they had immediately decontaminated themselves after the attack. However, the murder charges against them were dropped.

While a home-soil chemical attack such as this, or far worse, was truly the nightmare scenario, I cautioned the Abu Dhabi audience that it still remained unlikely at that time. I had no idea that, as I said these words, it had already happened.

As I walked off the stage and turned my phone back on, it suddenly came alive with a litany of beeps. Glancing down, I saw there were multiple missed calls from media organizations and intelligence contacts. *Probably just another attack in Syria,* I thought, having become almost used to the daily atrocities. But when I checked in with a contact in the intelligence world, I was told that it was Salisbury that had been attacked, my home town, where my wife and children lived. My jaw almost hit the floor.

News was still coming out in dribs and drabs but as my contact told me the details it already sounded extremely serious.

'The two victims are currently at Salisbury District Hospital,' he said. 'The doctor said they had to inject one of them with atropine over thirty times!'

'Christ . . .' I muttered. It would usually take a maximum of three atropine shots to treat someone subjected to a nerve agent. Thirty was virtually unheard of.

'Do they know what agent was used?' I asked.

'The doctor who treated them has actually worked on CBRN with the Territorials. He said it was unlike anything he had ever seen before.'

'What were the victims' symptoms?'

'They were found frothing at the mouth on a park bench, then they froze, almost like statues.'

'It sounds like a nerve agent,' I replied. 'Maybe sarin.' Yet even as I said this, I was aware that if thirty atropine shots had been used then it must have been either an extremely heavy dose of sarin or something far, far worse. And it seemed the doctor, who had some experience of CBRN, had already discounted the possibility that sarin had been used.

'What else do you know?' I asked, hoping that any information might help shed some light on the likely agent.

'The victims, father and daughter, are both Russian, and the father has a very interesting background.'

This was a bit of an understatement. Sergei Skripal was a former officer from Russia's GRU intelligence directorate, and had been a double agent in the 1990s before being arrested in Moscow in 2004. Following the Illegals Program spy swap in 2010, he had relocated to the UK and subsequently settled in Salisbury. However, he still had to keep an eye over his shoulder, as in 2006 the Russian parliament had passed a law permitting the extra-judicial killings abroad of those Moscow accused of 'extremism'. This effectively enabled enemies of the Russian state to be murdered by Russian state agents on foreign soil with absolute impunity.

The Russians certainly had previous form for this sort of thing, most notably the Georgi Markov incident in 1976, when the exiled Bulgarian writer had been pricked with an umbrella coated with ricin as he strolled across Waterloo Bridge. In more recent years, Alexander Litvinenko, another Russian defector to Britain, died after being poisoned with the radioactive material polonium-210 at London's Millennium Hotel. Investigators later concluded that the murder was a state-sponsored assassination.

'So we're thinking Russian agents are behind this?' I asked.

'Definitely,' my contact replied. 'We are looking into the identities and whereabouts of all known agents and any Russians who have recently entered the country.'

As he spoke, fragments of the puzzle started to come together in my mind. *This sounds like another state-sponsored Russian hit job . . . a nerve agent has clearly been used . . . but it sounds far more serious than any we have ever seen before . . . far more potent . . .*

'It could be Novichok,' I suddenly blurted out.

'What?'

I couldn't blame him for not having a clue what I was on about, such was the mystery and secrecy surrounding one of the world's most deadly agents.

Scientists in the Soviet Union first began to develop Novichok in the early 1970s. They claimed it was the deadliest nerve agent ever made, with some variants of it possibly being up to eight times more potent than VX. However, while there was plenty of talk and speculation about the agent, it was never actually used on the battle-field, so it was impossible for anyone in the West to analyse it. Yet in the late 1980s there had been a breakthrough.

In the late 1980s, Vladimir Pasechnik and other Russian scientists defected to the UK. They settled in Salisbury and shared their secrets at Porton Down. With this lifting of the lid on the Soviet chemical and biological weapon programme, which was based in Skihany, a few hundred miles from Moscow, we finally understood just how lethal Novichok could be. It was virtually undetectable and very persistent, lasting for years once it had been spread on to a surface. Most chillingly of all, just one molecule could kill millions of people. But as we had still not seen any evidence of it in action, some felt it might be more of a legend than an actual threat. If Novichok had been used in Salisbury, this would be unprecedented.

But I didn't have time to explain all of this to my contact, as another terrible thought suddenly struck me. 'The Skripals, where had they been before they were found?' I asked.

'All we know at this stage is that they had been at Sergei's home in Salisbury, then the Italian restaurant Zizzi, before they were found by members of the public in the Maltings area.'

This was extremely concerning. If it was Novichok, or even any other nerve agent, anything that the Skripals touched could be contaminated, not to mention the members of the public who found them, as well as the paramedics who initially treated them.

'You need to close off everywhere you know they've been and decontaminate those areas quickly,' I urged.

But it was already too late for some.

I later found that two of the police officers who had attended the Skripals' house soon after the attack required treatment for itchy eyes and wheezing, while one, Detective Sergeant Nick Bailey, was in a serious condition in hospital.

As it dawned on us how serious this incident could be, I cut the phone call short to speak to Julia. 'Julia, don't leave the house!' I breathlessly shouted as soon as she answered.

'What are you talking about?'

'Where are the children?' I asked, with no time to explain.

'Jemima is getting ready to go out and Felix is in the cinema in town.'

'Call him immediately, tell him to come home and tell him for Christ's sake don't touch anything.'

'Hamish, what on earth is the matter with you?'

It was only as I outlined the severity of the situation that Julia hung up and ensured that she and the children remained safe at home. Until the emergency teams had decontaminated the area, and had tracked all of the Skripals' movements, going into Salisbury was just too risky. Large parts of the country now know exactly how this feels following the outbreak of COVID-19, but coming into contact with Novichok would have been far more serious.

Returning to my hotel room, I quickly made arrangements to get the next flight back to the UK. As I hurriedly packed my case, thoughts ran through my head at a million miles an hour. I was not entirely surprised that something like this should happen in Salisbury. The town might appear to be a backwater on the surface but the presence of Porton Down on the outskirts attracted quite an array of characters. I was well aware that spies, double agents, scientists and intelligence agents were rife in the area. Many people in Salisbury did not realize that their next-door neighbour, who they happily greeted every morning, might actually have quite a backstory. I am sure that Sergei Skripal's neighbours knew nothing of his background. Indeed, there had been a number of occasions when I had visited a country pub for Sunday lunch only to find certain known individuals conspiring in a dark corner about issues that affected national security. Sometimes I had even been with these parties.

As I thought this, my phone continued to ring incessantly. I decided to turn it off. My contacts in the media were chasing me for a comment but for now I wanted to avoid talking. I didn't yet know all the details and I certainly didn't want to start a panic. Yet when I arrived in the UK the following morning, a full-scale panic was already underway. While the Prime Minister, Theresa May,

261

told Parliament, 'It's a nerve agent we haven't seen before,' the Chief Medical Officer advised everyone in Salisbury to burn any clothes they had been wearing that weekend. This led to my phone beeping even more frantically. Not just the media but friends and family too were all desperate for information, as were politicians, who had never had to deal with something like this before and didn't know what to tell their constituents.

Arriving home, I found it all very strange. Usually Salisbury was my sanctuary, a place where I could relax without the fear of chemical weapons. Now it was right at the heart of a major attack and it took a while to get my head around. I told my family to avoid Salisbury at all costs until the authorities had tracked all of the Skripals' movements. The risk of contamination was just too great. All it would take was for one of their fingertips to touch a contaminated surface and there was a good chance they would die. It seemed millions of others also got this message. Nearby Stonehenge usually hosts around 3.5 million American visitors every year, with many also visiting Salisbury Cathedral. After the attack most stayed away, which devastated local businesses.

While I wasn't actively involved in the investigation, this was certainly my area of expertise. As such, I was curious to get a better look at where the Skripals had been found, in the Maltings area of the city. I didn't expect to find any bombshell evidence but it was almost as if I had to see the site of the attack itself to actually believe it had happened. As I drove there, I was amazed at just how deserted the streets were. I barely saw a soul. Just as Britain was on COVID-19 lockdown for the spring and summer of 2020, Salisbury then was going through something very similar. There was hardly anyone walking the streets. It was clear that most people were terrified of this unknown, invisible enemy.

When I arrived at the Maltings, it looked like a scene from a war zone. Usually full of shoppers, the area was cordoned off, surrounded by police, while experts in hazmat suits collected further evidence. I was very surprised to see that the park bench where the Skripals had been found was still there. Though everyone was wearing PPE, the bench must surely have been contaminated and presented a danger. But at least we knew the bench was contaminated. The big question was: what else had been?

I feared that traces of the agent must be all over the town, lying in wait, just like a virus. I also feared more might be out there. I shook my head at the thought. The attack was so brazen, so reckless, that it almost defied belief. For over an hour, I stood in the bitter chill, watching flecks of snow slowly cover up the scene, as if a crisp white layer might somehow mask and suffocate the evil that had been perpetrated.

The next few days were a whirlwind. While I tried to give a calm and measured view of what we were dealing with, in interviews with the likes of the BBC and the *Guardian* at the site of the attacks, people were growing increasingly desperate for answers. I therefore said that in my opinion, based only on secondhand information at this point, it looked like Novichok could have been used. This really caused a storm but several days later it appeared my analysis had been correct.

First Theresa May, and then Porton Down, publicly confirmed that the agent used had been identified as one of the Novichok family of agents. This was also verified by the OPCW on 12 April. Indeed, weeks later, the head of the OPCW, Ahmet Üzümcü, informed the *New York Times* that about 50 to 100g of the nerve agent was thought to have been used in the attack. This indicated it was likely to have been created to be used as a weapon, and was enough to kill millions of people. It could have killed more people in Salisbury alone than COVID-19 has currently killed in the whole of the UK in mid 2020.

With panic and wild conspiracy theories flying around, I tried to make myself available on Twitter to answer any questions. However, it soon became apparent that I was being accused of spreading disinformation. The conspiracy theorists and 'useful idiots' were out in full force, as were Russian bots, who seized on any discrepancies to try to discredit the story that was now emerging. Thanks to poor communication lines, and plenty of ignorance, we actually made this very easy for them to do this.

While Theresa May outright pointed the finger at Russia for the assassination attempt, with this assessment backed up by twenty-eight other countries, the new head of Porton Down told Sky News that he wasn't sure who was responsible; to be fair to him it was not his place to comment on that and he probably hadn't even been briefed. Meanwhile, the Leader of the Opposition, Jeremy Corbyn, also appeared to be less than willing to name Russia as the likely culprit. Building on these seeds of disagreement and doubt, a major disinformation campaign on social media was soon underway, with Russian outlets posting at least sixty major pieces every day. One of their favourite theories suggested that this was a false flag attack and that the Novichok that had been used had come from nearby Porton Down. This totally ignored the fact that the UK hadn't actually manufactured nerve agents since the 1930s, apart from very small batches for research and testing. And this had certainly not been a small batch.

Such accusations were preposterous in any event. The UK had no motive for such an attack. Yet as I sought to correct this story, the trolls soon turned their attention on me. They raced to tear through my private and professional life, eager to access any information that could be used against me, which thankfully was not a lot. I did however start receiving threats in my direct messages, along the lines of 'You're next, DBG', which alarmed me after what had just happened, and especially knowing that Putin had already warned Dr Nott about my work. But rather than back away, I decided that we needed to confront this poisonous propaganda head on.

Speaking to friends in the intelligence world, as well as some individuals I knew to be close to the Skripals, I was encouraged to do all that I could to counter the fake narrative. For days I did the rounds on TV, spoke on the radio, did newspaper interviews and continued to answer questions on Twitter, ensuring that the record was set straight and the various conspiracies were shown to be totally ridiculous.

Meanwhile, the security services were hard at work investigating the crime. It appeared that the Novichok had been placed on the door handle of the Skripals' house, which Sergei and his daughter, Yulia, had both touched on their way out, as had Police Sergeant Nick Bailey, when he attended the property.

While the Skripals' house was being decontaminated by specialist teams, nine other sites were identified that could have also been contaminated. As such, 180 decontamination experts were deployed to remove vehicles and objects from any such sites, as well as to look for any further traces of the nerve agent. It took almost 18 months to decontaminate these areas, producing 13,000 bags of material and thirty-seven vehicles, which all needed to be destroyed and/ or buried in a secure location. Police Sergeant Bailey and his family also lost their home, which had to be demolished, while all of their clothing and possessions had to be destroyed, for fear they had been contaminated.

With Yulia and Sergei still fighting for their lives in hospital, Russia continued to deny any responsibility for the attack. It even denied manufacturing Novichok, which we knew to be total rubbish. Around this time the BBC contacted me. It had managed to obtain 1980s documentary footage from Skihany, the Russian chemical weapons factory, and asked if I would have a look at it before they aired it on *Newsnight*. I can't disclose how the BBC came to be in possession of the footage, but I knew this could be bombshell stuff. As they could not risk emailing such sensitive material, I visited the BBC headquarters in London, where I was shown the tape. Within that footage I found remarkable evidence that Novichok was being produced.

Yet as *Newsnight* revealed the story and the OPCW looked to investigate further, the Russians proceeded to level Skihany to the ground. All other evidence was also destroyed. It was an incredible act, and clearly indicated Russia's guilt, but even after this the 'truthers' still refused to accept that Russia was behind the attack. I suppose they just levelled their top chemical facility for the hell of it . . .

Sergei and Yulia slowly recovered and were both discharged from hospital by mid May, but the story was then to take a further incredible twist. On 20 June 2018, in the nearby town of Amesbury, a man by the name of Charlie Rowley found a perfume bottle in a charity shop bin. He subsequently gave it to his partner, Dawn Sturgess, who sprayed some of the 'perfume' on to her wrists. This was to prove fatal. Within fifteen minutes Sturgess had fallen ill and was to die in hospital three weeks later.

It transpired that the perfume bottle had contained Novichok. Many in the intelligence community felt it had probably been a spare bottle, which the Russian agents had thrown away after the initial attack. Again, there were enough molecules of Novichok in the bottle to have killed thousands. No one had any idea how long it had been in the charity shop bin but it was a miracle it had not smashed. The only positive about the discovery of the perfume bottle was that Porton Down at last had a good quality sample of Novichok to analyse.

Yet again, Russia tried to play dumb, while infecting the airwaves with more bile. But the Security Services and Counter Terrorist Police were at last closing in on those they believed were responsible. It had found that two Russians, travelling under the identities of Alexander Petrov and Ruslan Boshirov, had arrived in the UK the day before the attack. They had stayed at the City Stay Hotel in Tower Hamlets before travelling to Salisbury by train. As Theresa May announced that these two men were the prime suspects, thought to be members of Russia's GRU Intelligence Service, the hotel room where they had stayed was found to contain traces of Novichok.

The Russian news site Fontanka subsequently reported

that the numbers on leaked passport files for Petrov and Boshirov were only three digits apart. Incredibly, these fell in a range that also included the passport files for a Russian spy who had been expelled from Poland. This was a major blunder. It seemed to suggest that Petrov and Boshirov were spies, and it allowed any country to crosscheck passport data for any Russians requesting visas, to ascertain whether they might also be enemies of the state.

On 14 September 2018, the investigative website Bellingcat, as well as the Russian publication *The Insider*, noted that in Petrov's leaked passport files there was no record of a residential address or indeed any identification papers prior to 2009. This suggested that the name was an alias created that year. It was also found that Petrov's dossier was stamped 'Do not provide any information' and had the handwritten annotation 'SS', a common abbreviation in Russian for 'top secret'. On 15 September 2018, the Russian opposition newspaper *Novaya Gazeta* reported finding in Petrov's passport files a cryptic number that seemed to be a telephone number associated with the Russian Defence Ministry, most likely the Military Intelligence Directorate.

In the face of such damning evidence, I have to hand it to Putin and the Russians; they continued to come up with some quite laughable explanations for why these men had travelled to Salisbury. With no shame whatsoever, the men claimed in an interview that they had merely wanted to see the sights and purchase nutrition products. They also said that they 'maybe approached Skripal's house, but we didn't know where it was located', which seemed an incredible way of trying to explain their movements. Perhaps the biggest corker of them all was hearing them deny using Novichok, which they had allegedly transported in a fake perfume bottle, saying, 'Is it silly for decent lads to have women's perfume? The customs are checking everything, they would have questions as to why men have women's perfume in their luggage. We didn't have it.'

Soon afterwards, Bellingcat positively identified the man known as Ruslan Boshirov as the highly decorated GRU colonel Anatoliy Chepiga, who was made a Hero of the Russian Federation by decree of the President in 2014. Bellingcat also revealed the real identity of the suspect named by police as Alexander Petrov to be Dr Alexander Mishkin, also of the GRU. A third GRU officer present in the UK at this time was also identified as Denis Vyacheslavovich Sergeev, a graduate of Russia's Military Diplomatic Academy and believed to hold the rank of major general in the GRU. The pattern of his communications while in the UK indicated that he had liaised with superior officers in Moscow.

To date, no one has been brought to justice for this appalling and reckless crime. Indeed, it has been alleged since that in recent years Russia might have killed fourteen other so-called traitors on British soil. This includes the exiled oligarch Boris Berezovsky, who was found hanged at his home in 2013, as well as Scottish property developer Scot Young, who was found impaled on iron railings after he fell from his girlfriend's fourth-floor flat in West London. There have also been calls to reopen the investigation into the death of Russian scientist Vladimir Pasechnik, who informed Porton Down about biological weapons and Novichok, and died in mysterious circumstances in 2001, also in Salisbury.

In recent years a friend of mine also met a sad and tragic fate, with Russia again being accused of being involved. On 11 November 2019, James Le Mesurier, the co-founder of the White Helmets organization, was found dead on the street outside his apartment in Istanbul, seemingly after falling from his balcony. In the months before this James had been the target of some of the most disgusting propaganda I have ever seen. In a sustained smear campaign, Russian outlets and the usual 'useful idiots' accused the White Helmets of being an arm of Al-Qaeda and part of a 'George Soros conspiracy', in addition to other slanderous slurs that I have no interest in repeating here, such is their falsehood and barbarity.

It was clear that Assad and Putin very much viewed James and the White Helmets as the enemy, and when he was found dead in the street, after a fall from a balcony, this seemed very much to fit their modus operandi. However, Turkish investigators have since ruled out foul play, and James's wife has revealed that he had been recently diagnosed with serious hypertension and depression, perhaps due to all the false claims and threats against him. As such, it is believed he took his own life. Even if that is the case, I believe that the Russian and Syrian bots have blood on their hands for driving such a hateful campaign against a man who only wanted to help the Syrian people.

The events in Salisbury, and James's death in particular, were a real wake-up call for me. For a good few years I had found myself repeatedly smeared and threatened on social media, and I knew that Putin had warned David Nott about my work. It appeared that the Russian state has no misgivings about targeting those they believe are enemies, so I have had to take steps to protect myself, my home and my family.

The threat is very real, not just to myself but to plenty of others, and I can't but help think that the seeds for this were sown by the 2013 parliamentary vote against taking action in Syria. We were told at the time that a 'red line' had been crossed, and that if action wasn't taken then despots and terrorists would see chemical weapons as fair game. With no action taken, we have not only seen an explosion of chemical attacks across Syria and Iraq but we have now also witnessed attacks in the UK. Indeed, in recent months the rules have been pushed to breaking point, with ever more chemical attacks being seen around the globe . . .

18

Bending the Rules

The months that followed Salisbury were extremely concerning. With continued attacks in Syria, the UK's Joint Terrorism Analysis Centre changed the threat of a chemical attack from 'unlikely' to 'likely'. Everyone was on high alert, with government and city officials around the globe suddenly desperate to reduce the risk of a home-soil attack. Some asked for my help, but I cannot divulge much about my specific advice, due to security issues and client confidentiality. However, it was heartening to see officials finally wake up to the threat.

Intelligence suggested that the most likely places for such an attack were underground railway systems or sporting events. In particular, there was a real fear that the London Underground could be targeted by terrorists, as gas would sink through the system to the lowest levels. This would clearly cause chaos, and there was also a real risk that many more people would be hurt in their desperation to escape as panic set in.

Indeed, the fear of an attack, or the fear that you have been contaminated, can sometimes be as debilitating as the real thing, especially if it induces panic in a crowd. I remember once being with the BBC reporter John Simpson in Iraq, making a film for the 25th anniversary of the Halabja attack. While we were in Halabja, he became convinced that he was suffering from mustard gas poisoning. My subsequent tests proved that he had not been exposed to any agent but it showed that even an educated man like Simpson, who has spent a lot of time in war zones, was not aware of the symptoms and so worked himself into a panic. Of course, I could sympathize, being well aware of how the mere fear of a chemical attack could drive you to abject terror.

But an attack on the underground would have some very real consequences. Once the gas was released it would spread far and wide, with wind in the tunnels quickly pushing it to other stations, infecting platforms and stairwells. It was a nightmare scenario, with the potential for thousands of casualties. I was therefore happy to advise on how to avoid this and what to do if it should ever occur.

There were also real fears that the 2019 Superbowl between the LA Rams and New England Patriots would be a target. Tens of thousands of spectators were expected to cram into the Mercedes-Benz Stadium in Atlanta, Georgia, where intelligence indicated that a terror group might try to fly a drone over the crowd and release a chemical agent. When I heard this, I thought it almost sounded like something out of a Hollywood movie but it was very clear that this was a serious threat and could be easily achieved.

While a drone could release only relatively small and therefore not particularly lethal amounts of an agent, the chaos such an attack would cause would more than suffice. Indeed, sometimes the primary use of these weapons is to spread terror and this would certainly have achieved that, in front of a worldwide audience no less. Although I helped officials to plan for this scenario, I have no idea if any more came of it. It is, however, something that the organizers of all major sporting events must now consider.

However, rather than despots brazenly using outlawed weapons, such as Novichok or VX, the real issue lies with them bending the rules, without fear of any consequences. As we already know, Assad led the way when, shortly after apparently giving up his chemical stockpile to the UN, he utilized chlorine bombs to attack his own people. This was a significant moment. Not only was it the first time that a CWC signatory was found to be in breach but it also showed that even having given up their illegal chemical weapons, such as gas and nerve agents, countries could instead utilize toxic materials, such as chlorine, which lay in a legally grey area. Chlorine is cheap, certainly in comparison to the cost of developing nerve agents, and it can be bought in large quantities with no questions asked, as it is commonly used to treat water. It is, of course, only illegal when used as a weapon. Therefore, countries could legally build up this chemical stockpile and use it as a weapon when they saw fit, knowing that punishment for doing so was unlikely.

The very limited action taken against Assad for this appalling breach has legitimized other countries looking to take a similar course. For instance, while tear gas is legal under the Chemical Weapons Convention, when used within specified guidelines, it is illegal when used as a weapon. When riots broke out across Hong Kong in 2019, against plans to allow extradition to mainland China, tear gas was repeatedly used against protestors in enclosed areas, such as underground train stations. Because there is less air and fewer escape routes in these confined areas, the gas is far more potent. As a result, using tear gas in this manner is illegal. Nevertheless, despite global disapproval, Hong Kong officials continued to use the gas with wild abandon. It was reported that on 5 August alone the police fired 800 tear gas canisters at protestors, clearly using it as a weapon, and that during the riots as much as 88% of the population of Hong Kong might have been affected. This is an incredible statistic, and all this happened under the watching eyes of the world, who once more did nothing in response.

Similarly, the use of white phosphorus also isn't technically illegal under the Chemical Weapons Convention. Routinely held by militaries around the world, it is typically used in combat as a smokescreen in daytime or as an incendiary to light up an area at night. However, used as a weapon it is extremely dangerous, not to mention painful. Capable of burning at upwards of 4,800 degrees Fahrenheit, it sticks to skin like a jelly, causing horrific injuries. The natural reaction is to put water on it, but that actually makes things even worse. Smothering the affected area, to cut out the oxygen supply, is the only way to help settle it down.

Human Rights Watch has said about the effects of this incendiary: 'Victims who survive their initial injuries may suffer from intense pain, severe infections, organ failure and lowered resistance to disease . . . They may also suffer severe disfigurement and lifelong disability, psychological trauma, and an inability to reintegrate into society.'

Unsurprisingly, the use of white phosphorus as a weapon is considered to be illegal. However, countries that have been accused of using it in war zones in recent times, such as the USA and Israel, have claimed that they were using it merely for military purposes, such as for smoke screens, and that any subsequent injuries were purely accidental. It is, of course, very difficult to prove otherwise.

In October 2019, I received a phone call from a Kurdish friend.

'Hamish, they have attacked us with white phosphorous. What can we do?'

To my surprise, for once the finger was not pointed at Assad or Putin.

With the Kurds having enjoyed nearly six years of autonomy near the Turkish border, the Turkish government had become concerned at its growing influence. Inside its own borders, Turkey has for years tried to counter the threat of the Kurdistan Workers' Party, or PKK, a militant group that has regularly launched attacks across the country in the name of Kurdish nationalism. These attacks, and the Turkish government's countermeasures, have together killed tens of thousands over the past few decades. For Turkish President Recep Erdoğan, countering the PKK even took precedence over fighting ISIS.

When President Trump surprisingly announced that he would be pulling military support out of Syria in October 2019, he effectively left his Kurdish partners in the region at the mercy of Assad, Putin and Erdoğan. Sensing an opportunity to push the Kurds back from the border, as well as return some of the millions of Syrian refuges that had flooded into Turkey, Erdoğan wasted little time.

Launching an offensive into north-eastern Syria, dubbed Operation Peace Spring, Turkish forces unleashed air strikes and artillery barrages, aiming to establish a 32km buffer zone along the border, where it hoped to resettle one million Syrian refugees. The plan raised alarm in humanitarian circles, with advocates fearing that refugees would be forcibly returned to a conflict zone in violation of international law. This cut little ice with Erdoğan, who was determined to show strength, forcing hundreds of thousands of civilians to flee the fighting, while eighty civilians were killed. In the mayhem, Kurdish forces, who were guarding a network of ISIS prisons in the region, inadvertently allowed 100 dangerous prisoners to escape when the Turkish offensive forced them to abandon their posts. Yet the worst was still to come.

On 17 October 2019, air strikes and mortar shells rained down on the northern Syrian border town of Ras al-Ayn, which had been at the front line of Turkey's incursion against Kurdish forces. Local medics soon found that some of the victims' injuries were very unusual. Some were severely burnt, with a jelly-like substance stuck to their skin. Children who had been wounded in this manner subsequently required urgent evacuation to hospitals in Northern Iraq. It was from here that Kurdish officials, who I knew through my dealings with the Peshmerga, swiftly got in touch.

Informing me of the details, they sent me pictures of some of the victims' injuries, which made me wince. In one, a small child's flesh was severely burnt across its torso, appearing red raw. The child was lucky to be alive but would no doubt be disfigured for life. Sadly, the pictures appeared to back up the ever-growing evidence that white phosphorous had been used as a weapon.

'What should we do?' my Kurdish friend asked.

'You must take samples,' I replied, outlining all the procedures that must be followed.

As samples were collected at the hospital, I made some calls to see which organization would like to take them. To my surprise, it turned out that no one wanted to get involved, not the UN, Human Rights Watch or even the WHO. The standard answer most gave was that the use of white phosphorus was a grey area and therefore it was not for them to investigate. This was rubbish.

Article 1 of Protocol III of the CWC defines an incendiary weapon as 'any weapon or munition which is primarily designed to set fire to objects or to cause burn injury to persons through the action of flame, heat, or combination thereof, produced by a chemical reaction of a substance delivered on the target'. White phosphorous clearly fell under this definition. Article 2 of the same protocol prohibits the deliberate use of incendiary weapons against civilian targets, the use of air-delivered incendiary weapons against military targets in civilian areas, and the general use of other types of incendiary weapons against military targets located within concentrations of civilians without taking all possible means to minimize casualties.

Under this definition, it was quite clear that white phosphorous had been used as a weapon and was therefore illegal. In normal circumstances the likes of the OPCW would have been compelled to investigate, but wherever I turned I found myself up against a wall of silence.

'At least take the samples and look into it,' I repeatedly begged officials, but no one wanted to know. I believe that the real reason for this reluctance was the fear that Turkey, a member of the UN, would be implicated in the attack. This would not only cause deep embarrassment but would also be difficult to resolve. However, this should not have been the concern of the OPCW. All it should have concerned itself with was whether there had been a chemical attack, by a signatory country, which it was obligated to investigate. Sadly, the world is not so black and white, and to the OPCW this fell into a convenient grey area.

'I'm sorry,' I told my Kurdish friend. 'No one will take the samples.'

'Then what else can we do?' he asked.

'Nothing,' I replied, ashamed of what had happened. 'No one wants to know.'

It was a development which stunned us both. With the rules once more bent to suit various governments' needs, and no deterrent in place, it is surely only a matter of time before a far more serious incident occurs.

Thankfully, there is a somewhat happy ending to this terrible incident: I understand that all of the children who were injured in the attack are now as well as can be expected and some have even returned home. Still, the samples from the attack remain refrigerated for anyone who has the guts to take them.

19

The Future

As I write this, in the spring of 2020, the future of the world is very much on the precipice of change, if not downright revolution.

The events of the last eight years in Syria have for ever changed the world, opening the door to the use of chemical weapons almost as a matter of course. If military action had been taken in 2013, following the horrific attack in Ghouta, then I am certain that not only would that have prevented further attacks but also thousands of lives would have been saved. Since that failure, there have been an estimated sixty-two further chemical attacks in Syria.

In response, the UN has been hamstrung by Russia's constant veto and the OPCW has been unable to enter the country to conduct a thorough investigation, not to mention refer Assad, Putin and their thugs to the International Criminal Court. It is clear that things must change. Never again can such atrocities be allowed to go unchallenged, in the face of such damning evidence.

The Future

With the UN and the OPCW proving to be a blunt tool, and the West refusing to take action, this has only encouraged the likes of Assad, Putin and Kim Jong-un to assassinate their enemies with prohibited chemical weapons, on foreign soil no less. It is outrageous that such deadly weapons, with the capability to kill thousands, if not millions, have been used in civilian areas to murder people and that those responsible have not faced any real consequences. Where is the deterrent to stop them performing such hazardous and reckless actions again?

As I write, the Syrian civil war finally appears to be coming to a close, as the last opposition-held area, Idlib, looks set to fall. With the region being bombarded regularly by Syrian, Russian and Iranian warheads, a terrible humanitarian crisis is unfolding. Hundreds of thousands of men, women and children are trying to cross the border to escape annihilation, but as mentioned in the previous chapter, Turkey will no longer take any more refugees, having taken 4 million already. These poor souls are therefore trapped in the most appalling conditions, after a terrible winter followed by a poor spring, with little food, medicine, clothes or warmth. Most live in tents, with almost all infrastructure having been destroyed, all the while being bombed on a regular basis, and hospitals are still being targeted.

The world has left the Syrian people to this fate, in the hope that this nightmare will soon be over. Millions will have died or been displaced from their homeland, while an entire country has been totally destroyed, all to keep one man in power. My only hope is that, thanks to the evidence that has been collected by people like Houssam Alnahhas, who bravely risked his life to prove that there had been a chemical attack in Talmenes, Assad and his evil henchmen will one day face justice in an international court. On that day, I know Houssam will confidently take the witness stand, look this pathetic coward in the eye, and, thanks to his evidence, ensure that Assad spends the rest of his wretched life behind bars.

Indeed, in April 2020, the OPCW released its latest and most hard-hitting report yet, accusing the Syrian regime of launching sarin and chlorine attacks on the town of Ltamenah in late March 2017. The evidence is now undeniable and mounting up. Enjoy your victory while it lasts, Assad, because soon enough you will be paying a very high price.

Yet while the war in Syria comes to a bitter end, the world is currently united in facing a common enemy: COVID-19. Sweeping the globe in a matter of months, this flu-like virus has already caused hundreds of thousands of deaths and shut down entire countries. It is unlike anything we have seen in our lifetime.

The virus is believed to have originated from Wuhan, China, although how this happened is still open to conjecture. It may have somehow been transmitted from an animal to a human at Huanan Seafood Wholesale Market, where seafood and wild and farmed animal species are sold. However, there is also a theory that this virus might have originated from the Wuhan Institute of Virology, China's only biosafety level-4 facility, which keeps more than 1,500 strains of deadly viruses and specializes in research into the most dangerous pathogens, in particular into viruses carried by bats. For now, it is difficult to say how valid this theory may be, but as I write yet more information is emerging that suggests this certainly warrants further investigation.

Indeed, the *Washington Post* has reported that in early 2018 the US Embassy in Beijing sent two official warnings back to Washington about inadequate safety at the Wuhan lab, including that it was conducting risky studies on pathogens in the coronavirus family in bats. Moreover, after the COVID-19 outbreak began, various reports claimed that officials at the lab destroyed virus samples, erased early reports and suppressed academic papers.

In any event, no matter where the virus came from, we know it is highly contagious and spreading like a biological weapon (although I must make it absolutely clear that I do not believe it was man-made). However, as tackling the pandemic bears some similarities to tackling a biological attack, my experience in CBRN has at least been of some help. While I have advised health boards on decontamination and the use of Personal Protective Equipment, now familiar to all as PPE, I have also advised on setting up Project Nightingale, which turned the ExCel Centre in London into a coronavirus-specific hospital. I have also been in talks with various organizations about the potential for using PCR machines for virus testing, in the hope that each machine might be able to quickly perform thousands of tests.

However, I have also had to once more turn my attention to Syria. As you might imagine, refugee camps, where millions of people are cramped together, are the perfect breeding ground for coronavirus. Yet though there are reports of the virus rampaging through the camps, and the medics having a only handful of ventilators available, Assad has refused to provide help, even refusing to admit that the virus is present in Syria, a belief that is in direct conflict with the views of the UN and WHO. It is clear that he has no intention of helping any of the refugees in Idlib and is no doubt hoping that the virus will wipe them out. Rather than having to use chemical weapons, he can sit back and let the virus do the dirty work for him. This is an atrocity that has the potential to unfold at a biblical scale in the coming weeks and months – and if Assad stands back and allows this to happen, every death will be on his hands.

Knowing this appalling situation, I have tried to help as best I can. With medical staff desperately requiring PPE, I have sent as many protection hoods to the camps as I can get my hands on, so that medics can treat victims without the fear of being contaminated by the virus. I also recently received a call from a charity worker based in the Rukban refugee camp near the Jordanian border. Five pregnant women, who were in desperate need of C-sections, couldn't be transferred to hospitals in Jordan, due to COVID-19 and the borders being closed. With no medical facilities in Rukban, the situation was desperate and I was asked if there was any way I could help. I wasn't quite sure what I could do, but after speaking to the Right Honourable James Cleverly, MP, Minister for the Middle East, he quickly contacted American special forces who were based at the nearby Tanf Airbase. Agreeing to do all that they could, soon afterwards they managed to airlift the women to their base, where a nurse was able to perform a C-section on one of them, with a US surgeon advising over Skype. I am told that both mother and baby are in rude health, a little ray of sunshine in these difficult times.

As for myself, I have again had to face some health issues. In July 2019, while I was in Syria running a refresher CBRN course for doctors, I received a phone call from my own doctor back home. Just before I had flown out, I had undergone a biopsy after tests had shown my prostate-specific antigen (PSA) levels to be slightly high, so this call was not entirely unexpected.

'I'm afraid your biopsy is positive,' the doctor told me. 'You have a grade-6 tumour in your prostrate.'

I was well aware that prostate cancer was the biggest

killer in men my age, so this seemed dreadful news. However, the doctor somewhat settled my nerves by telling me that grade-6 tumours grow very slowly, so for now, at least, they would continue to monitor my PSA levels before deciding what to do next.

I must admit, this news still left me a little shaken, and I was certainly feeling sorry for myself. However, as I slouched in a seat in the corridor, presumably looking very miserable, I caught sight of a young boy out of the corner of my eye. He was no more than two years old and had countless tubes and wires coming out of him, hooked up to some sort of machine. As I looked at him, I saw he had no legs and only one arm. I later learnt he had been blown up in an air attack by the Syrian regime two weeks earlier, losing all his family except his mother, who now sat by his side.

As the boy looked up at me, there was a twinkle in his eye and his face started to twitch, the edge of a smile appearing. I stared back, a small grin also appearing on my own face, entranced by this young boy. Suddenly he burst into a huge grin, showing his pearly white teeth. It almost bought me to tears. Here I was feeling sorry for myself, when this young child, after all he had been through, could still smile in the face of terrible adversity. I felt the need to do something and reached into my pockets. All I had was my passport and a fifty-dollar bill, so I gave his mother the money and wished them both luck.

The Future

While I continue to be treated for prostate cancer, and my dicky heart is always at the back of my mind, this young boy's example has ensured that I certainly haven't slowed down and am as busy as ever. Through my own experiences, and having witnessed so much death, I am very aware that our time on this earth is precious, and therefore mean to make every moment count. When you are aware that you have a heart condition that could instantly turn out the lights then there is no other way to live. There could be no tomorrow so today has to count.

In recent months, I have joined the Engineer Logistic Staff Corps, which is a group of experts who provide advice to the MOD on a pro bono basis. With the increasing CBRN threat, my current task is to advise the MOD on the formation of a new CBRN Regiment, after it was disbanded in December 2011, in an attempt to save £129m over the following decade. This was, of course, shortly after the financial crash, when the government was looking to cut costs wherever it could, but I found this to be a step too far, as it could have been a real national security issue. While some of its capabilities were taken on by the RAF, it has been clear in recent years that we have sorely missed a dedicated CBRN Regiment. I'm thankful to now have the opportunity to advise on how we can get this vital military arm up and running once more.

Meanwhile, my time at Avon has also come to an end, as I have been asked to be a visiting fellow at Magdalene

College, Cambridge, studying humanitarian intervention. This is, of course, a tremendous – and unexpected – opportunity, particularly for someone who flunked almost all of their school and university exams. Nevertheless, I am looking forward to helping to educate and inspire the next generation of experts; they will no doubt be needed in the coming years. It amazes me that not that long ago I was begrudgingly being sent to complete a chem bio diploma at Shrivenham, and now I will be lecturing at one of the world's most prestigious universities. It just goes to show that once you find your passion, anything is possible.

And that certainly goes for Julia and me. We are still very much the happy couple and will shortly be celebrating our twenty-eighth wedding anniversary. It's amazing to think that she has somehow put up with me, and my adventures, for all that time. I know I'm sometimes not an easy person to live with, but I couldn't have done it without her. As well as coming to Germany with me at the start of my career, so that I could be a Tankie, in more recent years she has been a rock, as the events in Syria sometimes threatened to overwhelm me. There is no better partner I could have asked for on this journey.

I probably still don't speak about emotions as often as I should but I'm working on it, and writing this book has certainly helped me work through some things. I feel more positive about the future than I have for a long time, which is really saying something in these dark times. I still have a raging fire in my belly to make a difference, and just in the last few days I received a call from my good friend Dr David Nott.

'Hamish, I'm going to Syria. Do you want to come with me to train some of the staff on PPE and decontamination for COVID?'

At this I looked at Julia, shaking her head, exasperated but already knowing my answer.

'Count me in,' I replied, eager for the next challenge.

If you can force your heart and nerve and sinew
To serve your turn long after they have gone,
And so hold on where there is nothing in you
Except the Will that says to them: 'Hold on!'

From 'If—', by Rudyard Kipling

Appendix

Surviving a Chemical or Biological Attack

Since the Salisbury attack, I have been struck by just how concerned the public are that these events might be repeated and by the lack of practical advice that is out there.

Compared to countries such as South Korea, we are certainly lagging behind. On the Korean tube they display instructions for people to follow should a chemical attack occur, and escape hoods are provided in stations. South Koreans are always on high alert in case of an attack from their neighbour in the north, but having such information in front of people daily not only prepares them but also makes them feel less afraid.

I feel this is important. Rather than engage in scaremongering, as some like to do when discussing chemical attacks, clear and concise advice should be readily available, to demystify some of the myths. Indeed, when I first attended the chem bio course in Shrivenham much of what I knew of chemical weapons had come from the movie *The Rock*, in which VX is seen melting someone's face. This is, of course, total rubbish but no doubt most people who have seen the film will now believe this to be true. However, one of the very few benefits of the COVID-19 outbreak is that far more people in the UK now carry PPE with them, such as protective gloves and face masks, which would be invaluable in the event of a chemical attack.

But in case you should ever be unfortunate enough to find yourself in the middle of such an attack (and please remember there is still very little chance of this happening), here are some straightforward tips to help you identify the agent, how to react and what treatment to seek.

CHLORINE

Smell and sight: Typically used as a gas, a green and yellow cloud is usually seen, which will smell like strong bleach or like a swimming pool.

Exposure: Chlorine cannot penetrate your skin but can be lethal if inhaled, especially for children. Therefore as long as your mouth and nose are protected, you should not be contaminated.

Symptoms: If the gas is inhaled, symptoms can include difficulty breathing, coughing, sneezing, nose irritation, burning sensations and throat irritation. In more serious cases there may be skin or eye irritation, chemical burns, nausea, vomiting or headaches.

Appendix

Advice: Get to higher ground as soon as you can, as the gas is heavier than air and therefore sinks to the floor quickly. The gas will also travel with the wind so it is important that you try to get upwind as soon as you can. If you can't get to higher ground or escape the cloud, an item of clothing, soaked in urine and then placed over your nose and mouth, is a very effective way to neutralize the gas before it enters your respiratory system. It is also important to remove clothes and to wash the chlorine off your skin as soon as possible.

Treatment: Most people with mild to moderate exposure generally recover fully in three to five days without requiring further treatment. Those who have received a heavy dose typically require oxygen and to have their lungs flushed with a bronchodilator, to decrease resistance in the respiratory airway and increase airflow to the lungs.

Persistence: Chlorine is not persistent and will evaporate quickly.

MUSTARD AGENT aka GAS

Smell and sight: Mustard gas usually smells like garlic, onions or mustard but it sometimes has no odour at all, while the gas itself will appear yellow or brown.

Exposure: Unlike chlorine, mustard gas can cause injury either by inhalation or by penetrating the skin. Therefore just covering your mouth and nose will not ensure protection.

Appendix

Symptoms: After being exposed, symptoms might not appear immediately and can take days to develop. Typical symptoms include red and itchy skin, painful yellow blisters, irritated eyes, blindness, runny nose, sneezing, sinus pain, sore throat, shortness of breath, coughing, abdominal pain, fever, nausea and vomiting. These symptoms can last for ten days.

Advice: As with chlorine, it is important to get to higher ground and upwind. If possible, avoid breathing in the gas or allowing your skin to be exposed to it. If you are exposed, you will need to get the mustard off your body as quickly as possible. You should remove your clothes, preventing others from touching them, and wash any exposed parts of your body with clean water. Eyes should also be flushed with water for 5 to 10 minutes. Due to the delayed reaction you might feel unaffected for a few hours after the attack but it is still important that you seek medical attention.

Treatment: There is no antidote for mustard gas exposure but it is not usually fatal. Most treatment involves further attempts to clean any exposed areas.

Persistence: Mustard gas can be very persistent, lasting for months under average weather conditions; in the cold it can freeze and persist for years. I tested some cellars in Halabja for mustard gas in 2012, twenty-four years after the attack, and still found microscopic traces of the agent. It is therefore vital that any exposed areas are avoided, and that they are decontaminated quickly to prevent cross contamination.

Appendix

ANTHRAX (biological pathogen)

Smell and sight: While typically mixed with white powder, anthrax spores are so small that they are invisible and have no smell.

Exposure: Anthrax is usually inhaled but it can also penetrate the skin through lacerations or abrasions, no matter how minor.

Symptoms: Symptoms can vary depending on whether the spores were inhaled or penetrated the skin. However, symptoms can take up to seven days to appear after exposure.

In cases where the skin has been penetrated, symptoms include raised itchy bumps that resemble an insect bite. This can develop into a fluid blister and then an ulcer with a black centre.

In cases where the anthrax has been inhaled, initial symptoms may resemble an influenza-like illness with sore throat, mild fever, muscle aches and fatigue. These symptoms may progress to severe breathing problems and shock, with meningitis frequently developing.

Advice: Unless you are the victim of a visible white powder attack, it will be difficult to know whether you have even been infected for hours or days afterwards, when you would normally expect to display symptoms.

Appendix

If, however, you are aware that you have been subjected to anthrax via an envelope attack, these are the steps I recommend you follow:

- Do not shake or empty the contents.

- Do not carry the package or envelope, show it to others or allow others to examine it.

- Put the package or envelope on a stable surface. If any contents have spilled, do not sniff, touch, taste or look closely at it.

- Alert others in the area. Leave the area, closing any doors behind you and take action to prevent others from entering the area. If possible, shut off the ventilation system.

- Wash hands with soap and water to prevent spreading potentially infectious material to your face or other areas of the skin. Seek additional instructions for exposed or potentially exposed persons.

- If at work, notify a supervisor, a security officer or law enforcement official. If at home, contact the local law enforcement agency.

- If possible, create a list of people who were in the room or area when the suspicious letter or package was recognized and a list of people who may have handled the letter or package. Give the lists to both the local public health authorities and law enforcement officials.

Appendix

Treatment: Due to the delayed reaction you might not be aware you have been subjected to anthrax until you develop the above symptoms. If treatment is sought early enough, administering antibiotics is usually very successful. However, as most victims don't know they have been infected until it is too late, there is a 75% death rate for those who have inhaled anthrax and not sought treatment in time.

Persistence: Anthrax spores are very persistent and have been known to last for decades on exposed surfaces. It is therefore vital that any exposed areas are professionally decontaminated.

SARIN (nerve agent)

Smell and sight: While sarin is a liquid, it is usually dispersed as a clear and odourless gas and so is hard to detect.

Exposure: Sarin can be inhaled as well as penetrate the skin, and also contaminates food, water and clothing.

Symptoms: Unlike anthrax, victims of sarin do not suffer from a delayed reaction after exposure. Victims usually develop symptoms within 10 minutes, which can prove fatal. Typical symptoms include: pinpoint pupils, coughing, tight chest, vomiting, diarrhoea, confusion, drowsiness, headache, weakness, sweating, muscle spasms, loss of consciousness, convulsions, paralysis.

Appendix

Advice: If you are aware that sarin has been used, it is important to get to higher ground and reach fresh air as quickly as possible. All clothing should be removed and the entire body washed with soap and water. Do not remove clothing over the head – cut it off instead. As infected clothing is contagious, and can release sarin for about 30 minutes after exposure, potentially infecting yourself or others, this should be sealed in a bag as quickly as possible. Eyes should be rinsed with plain water for 10 to 15 minutes if they are burning or if vision is blurred.

Treatment: It is essential that medical care is sought as quickly as possible, where atropine and pralidoxime might be administered to reverse the effects. However, both antidotes must be given within about 10 minutes of exposure in order to be effective. Therefore, time is of the essence.

Persistence: Sarin is thankfully a relatively non-persistent agent and evaporates at about the same rate as water. High temperature, humidity, wind and moisture can increase the rate of evaporation.

VX (nerve agent)

Smell and sight: VX is an odourless and tasteless oily liquid that is amber in colour. It can also be dispersed as gas if it is heated to very high temperatures.

Appendix

Exposure: VX can penetrate the skin or can be inhaled by breathing in its mist.

Symptoms: As with sarin, victims may not know they have been exposed to VX because it has no odour. Depending on the dosage, victims might display symptoms immediately or within a few hours. These typically include: blurred vision, chest tightness, confusion, cough, diarrhoea, drooling, excessive sweating, drowsiness, eye pain, headache, nausea, vomiting and/or abdominal pain, rapid breathing, pinpoint pupils, convulsions, loss of consciousness, paralysis and respiratory failure.

Advice: If you believe VX has been dispersed, you should quickly leave the area, get to higher ground and find fresh air. Clothing should be removed – cut off clothes that would normally be pulled over the head – and then safely disposed of. The entire body should be washed with soap and water, and medical attention sought as quickly as possible.

Treatment: The victim is usually decontaminated with household bleach and water before being injected with atropine and pralidoxime. In the case of convulsions, an injected sedative/antiepileptic such as diazepam is administered.

Persistence: VX is extremely persistent and in storage can last for as long as fifty years. It is therefore vital that all contaminated areas are urgently decontaminated.

Appendix

The key points to take away from all of this are:

GET HIGH

GO AGAINST THE WIND

DON'T PANIC

TAKE OFF CLOTHES

WASH

SEEK MEDICAL TREATMENT

If you bear these in mind, then should you be unfortunate enough to be caught in a chemical attack, you will have a far higher chance of survival.

Acknowledgements

Firstly, thanks go to James Leighton, the wordsmith who has put my pages of notes and hours of rambling stories into a coherent narrative. A singularly impressive skill from a great writer at the top of his game.

The brilliant author Damien Lewis set me off on this trip and persuaded me that my story is one people will want to hear. Thank you so much to him for his time and advice, and for introducing me to my agent, Gordon Wise of Curtis Brown. Publishing is an alien world to me, which Gordon effortlessly guided me through. He exudes confidence and his position at the top of the industry is well-founded.

Gordon and I had a really interesting round of discussions with various publishers, but Fiona Crosby and all the team at Headline stood out from the beginning for me. Their continual can-do attitude, especially during COVID-19, has been inspiring. Thanks go to Mari Evans, Rosie Margesson, Joe Yule, Georgie Polhill, Becky Bader, Chris Keith-Wright, Izzy Smith, Nathaniel Alcaraz-Stapleton, and many more involved behind-the-scenes.

There have been many people who have supported me along the way, but I must single out Professor David Nott, a legend, who has given me so much help and encouragement.

Acknowledgements

I am an imposter when people mention us in the same breath! Elly Nott's support has also been most welcome and I'm looking forward to working closely with her at Cambridge next year.

To my many Syrian friends, most especially Dr Ghanem Tayara of UOSSM, I owe a great debt of gratitude and I will continue to work with them as long as I can. The Iraqi Kurds, who have suffered so much through the ages, have a special place in my heart too, especially the men and women of the Peshmerga who did so much to defeat ISIS in Iraq.

My gratitude goes to the many people named in the book who have given their permission and helped me to remember some of the facts, often dimmed over time. There are many more people that I cannot thank openly, be they in the shadows or wherever, but they all know who they are and what part they play.

In writing my memoir we have had to tread a tightrope, especially with my military career, not to give up information of use to our adversaries. I'm indebted to my Regimental colleague and friend Lt Col Tim How and all at the Directorate of Defence Communications for their really useful comments and advice.

And, of course, the greatest thanks go to 'Champ', Mrs DBG, for putting up with me for twenty-eight years.